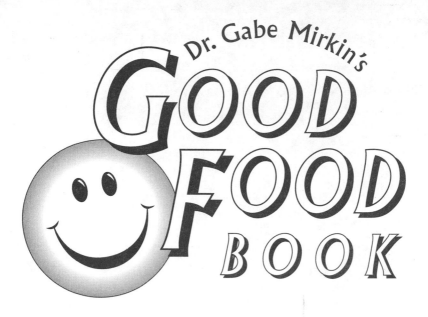

Dr. Gabe Mirkin's GOOD FOOD BOOK

Live Better and Longer with Nature's Best Foods

Includes 100 Delicious, Healthy Recipes

D0036593

By Gabe Mirkin, M.D. and Diana Mirkin

Nothing in this book is intended to replace the advice of a qualified health
professional. If your doctor or registered dietician have given you instructions
that contradict the information in this book, discuss your particular situation
with him or her and follow the advice given by your health care provider.

Copies are available at quantity discounts when used to promote products or
services. For information, call 1-800-420-4726 or write to:
LINX, Corp., PO Box 613, Great Falls, VA 22066 USA

FEATURES

1. INTRODUCTION

A healthy diet supplies enough calories (but not too many) to meet your energy needs, plus all the protein, essential fats, vitamins, minerals, phytochemicals and fiber you need to stay healthy and help to prevent diseases.

To get everything your body needs from the food you eat, without taking in too many calories, MOST of your food should be full of nutrients. This can be hard when you are bombarded with "junk" foods that are loaded with calories and have very little other nutritional value.

This is not another diet book – it's an explanation and listing of all the nutrient-rich foods available in your supermarket and restaurants. Use it to help you make good food choices.

THE 80%—20% GOAL

A reasonable goal for anyone who wants a healthy diet is to try to fill 80% of your plate with foods from this list – fruits, vegetables, whole grains, beans and other seeds; what you do with the remaining 20% is entirely up to you.

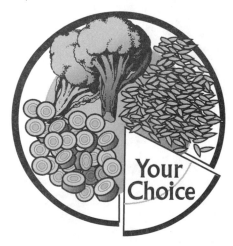

SPECIAL SITUATIONS

Almost everyone can use these food lists and the 80%-20% goal. Chapter 5 for extra helpful tips if you are:

- **Diabetic**
- **Need to lower cholesterol or blood pressure**
- **Want to lose or gain weight**
- **Pregnant or nursing**

You'll also find tips for seniors, children, active teens and athletes; and people who eat in restaurants often or are just too busy.

PLEASE NOTE: This book is not intended to replace the advice of a qualified medical professional. If material in this book in any way contradicts what your physician or registered dietician tells you, discuss it and follow his or her instructions for your specific situation.

STAY CLOSE TO NATURE

The human race evolved on the foods that were available – plants and animals that were gathered and hunted. Our bodies adapted to use the nutrients available in these foods. In the last few thousand years, humans learned to cultivate foods to make their supply more reliable and convenient, but domesticated plants and animals still contain all the nutrients of their wild predecessors. The healthiest diet for humans contains a wide variety of plants; usually has whole grains and beans as the staple foods (the ones that supply the most calories) and may include meat, fish and dairy products in smaller amounts.

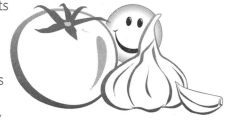

Our ancestors began to create nutritional problems when they found that they could store foods longer, make them easier to prepare and more tasty by removing the parts that spoiled quickest and eating only the starch, sugar or extracted oils. They discarded the minerals, vitamins, phytochemicals and omega-3 fatty acids that are found in the germ of seeds, creating serious deficiencies. We now have laws requiring some of these nutrients to be added back in to commercial flours, but that has only corrected the most obvious problems.

For most of human history the struggle has been to get enough food, so the survivors were those best equipped to cope with deprivation and scarcity. For most North Americans today, the problem is too much food that is too cheap, too convenient and too tasty to resist. We are bombarded with huge portions of sweet drinks, fried foods, bakery products made from white flour and other "empty" foods. It's all too easy to meet your whole day's calorie needs (2000-3000 calories or even more) with foods made almost entirely of sugar, white flour and added fats.

You may be able to exist on an unhealthy diet for a while, even for many years, but eventually it will catch up with you. Diabetes, heart problems, obesity, many cancers and other health problems are caused by or linked to unhealthy diets. If you are already in trouble, it's never too late to make dietary changes to help to reverse your health problems. It's far better to start early and eat in a healthy way all your life.

The next several pages summarize the nutrients you should get from your food, and their functions.

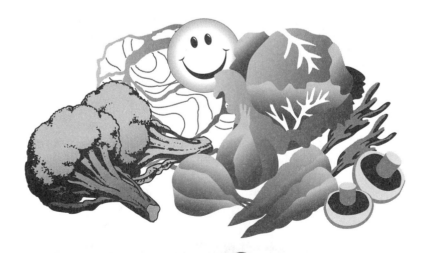

2. WHY YOU NEED FOOD

Plants make all the energy they need from sunlight and air, with the help of water and minerals they draw up through their roots. We can't do that; we get our energy and raw materials from food. We eat plants, and animals who have eaten plants, to get all the nutrients our bodies need to grow, reproduce and stay healthy. Human nutrition is fascinating; if you'd like to know more than this quick summary, check some of the resources on page 196. Here's what we need to get from our food:

ENERGY

Everything you do and all of the functions of your body use energy. Our only source of energy is the food we eat. Most people use between 1500 and 2500 calories (units of energy) per day.

If the food you eat contains more calories than you burn, you store the excess as fat. Any time you eat fewer calories than you need for your daily activities, your body uses your stored fat for energy.

Your body can use protein, carbohydrates or fats from your food for energy.
> **FAT**=9 calories per gram
> **CARBOHYDRATES**=4 calories per gram
> **PROTEIN**=4 calories per gram

These three macronutrients — protein, carbohydrates and fats — also have other important functions. A healthy diet contains enough, but not too much, of each.

PROTEIN

Protein supplies the building blocks for all the tissues and functions in your body. These building blocks, amino acids, are used
to make new cells and all the enzymes and other chemicals your
body requires to function. Your body uses 22 different amino acids,
and nine of those must come from the food you eat. These are
called the essential amino acids. Your body can make the remaining
amino acids from the essential nine.

Most people need between 50 and 75 grams of protein a day.
Protein deficiency is virtually unheard of in North America, since
any reasonably varied diet will give you plenty. Too much protein
can be a concern, so before you decide to follow a fad high-protein
diet or take protein supplements, understand that your body cannot store excess protein. Any unused protein is burned for energy
or stored as fat, and this process can stress the kidneys or liver and
may pull calcium out of bones.

Meat, fish and dairy products are good sources of protein, since
they contain all of the nine essential amino acids. However, meat
and dairy products also contain a lot of saturated fat, so most people (except competitive athletes and very active young people)
should choose skim milk products and limit or avoid meats. For
everyone except strict vegetarians, we recommend 2-3 servings of
seafood a week, and 2-3 servings of skim milk dairy products a day.
If you are lactose intolerant, you can use vegetarian milk substitutes
(see page 61.)

Most plants contain some, but not all of the essential amino acids.
Strict vegetarians can get all the amino acids they need from whole
grains and beans. The beans may contain only seven of the essential
nine, but the grains will have the other two. You do not need to do
special combinations at each meal to get
"complete protein"; just eat a
variety of grains, beans
and other vegetarian
choices each week.

FATS

Fats are the most concentrated sources of calories, so high-fat foods are good sources of energy. You need some fat (the essential fatty acids), but for most people, it's hard not to eat too much fat. Fatty foods are everywhere, because manufacturers know that fat makes food taste good.

There are two major categories called saturated and unsaturated fats. When you take in more calories than your body needs, saturated fats raise cholesterol and increase risk for heart attacks.

Polyunsaturated fats are healthful as long as they are left in their natural state and not converted to partially hydrogenated fats. The "good" fats are liquid at room temperature. They are found all plants and in seafood. Unsaturated fats are further classified into omega-3, omega-6 and more, depending on their chemical structure. Omega-3 polyunsaturated fats are particularly healthful because they help to prevent clotting and swelling that increase your risk for heart attacks and cancers.

The essential fatty acids (omega-3's and omega-6's) are fats that your body cannot assemble from other fats, so you must get them in your food. Omega 6's are abundant in vegetable oils, and most people get plenty. But Omega-3's, found in seeds, whole grains and seafood, may be lacking unless you make a special effort to eat these foods. The Omega-3's are the least stable of the fats (they turn rancid quickly when exposed to air, light or heat), so they are not found in most processed foods.

Unless you burn huge amounts of calories, limit or avoid fats that are solid at room temperature – the saturated fats found in butter, meats and high-fat dairy products. We believe that everyone should try to avoid partially hydrogenated vegetable oils, found in margarine, cookies, crackers and hundreds of other processed foods (see below). Several studies link these chemically altered vegetable oils with increased rates of heart attacks and cancers.

The best fats are those you eat IN parts of plants – whole grains, beans, nuts and other seeds. When you eat corn, olives, wheat berries, soybeans, sunflower seeds or peanuts instead of their extracted oils, you get all the fiber, vitamins, minerals and phytochemicals nature packages with the fat, not just the calories.

People who need to lose weight should avoid all added fats (butter, margarine, oils, and processed foods made with any of these ingredients). They also need to be cautious with nuts and snack seeds, which are packed with nutrients but are so tasty that it's hard to stop with a reasonable portion size (1-2 tablespoons.)

HOW TO AVOID PARTIALLY HYDROGENATED FATS:

The only way to cut back or eliminate partially hydrogenated fats (the source of trans fats) from your diet is to read the label of virtually every processed food you buy. Scan through the list of ingredients and if it contains the words "partially hydrogenated", put it back on the shelf.

It's much harder when you eat out, because you have no way to tell what's going on in the kitchen. Fast food restaurants and chains use a lot of pre-prepared (read "frozen") foods that they re-heat for you. These are usually loaded with partially hydrogenated fats. You're safer at restaurants that prepare your food from scratch. Asian restaurants are good bets: they may not be low-fat, but they use oils, not margarine or shortening. Most French or continental restaurants (read "expensive") use huge amounts of butter, better than trans fats but not great if you're trying to lose weight or control cholesterol. Italian, Greek, Spanish and other Mediterranean restaurants tend to use olive oil, a healthier choice.

CARBOHYDRATES

Plants store energy in the form of carbohydrates (sugars and starches — the products of photosynthesis). When you eat carbohydrates, they are quickly broken down into the sugar molecules you burn for energy. You can only store about 12 hours worth of sugar in your liver and your bloodstream; any excess is stored as fat, which can be broken back down into sugar for later use.

Carbohydrates contain single sugars or combinations of sugars. Glucose is an example of a single sugar. Sucrose or common table sugar is a double sugar. Starch contains thousands of sugar molecules bound together, while fiber contains millions of sugars bound together so tightly that your body cannot break them down. Only single sugars can pass from your intestines into your bloodstream. Double, triple, other combinations of sugars and starches must first be split into single sugars before they can be absorbed. These reactions occur so rapidly in your intestines that most starches cause rises in blood sugar that are not much lower than those of single sugars.

In nature, sugars and starches are always paired with vitamins, minerals, phytochemicals and fiber. Our ancestors, in their long quest for food that stores better, tastes better and is easier to prepare, learned to remove the starches and sugars from the other nutrients, giving us the first "junk" food. Food manufacturers in the twentieth century perfected the process of taking highly nutritious plants and turning them into all kinds of nutritionally empty products – soft drinks, juices, cookies, crackers, chips, bakery products, sugar coated breakfast cereals, the list goes on and on. We now have endless choices of food loaded with sugar, white flour and other refined carbohydrates. Most of the vitamins, minerals, phytochemicals and fiber have been stripped away.

We now have laws that require manufacturers to add some of the B vitamins back into flour, and vitamins and minerals are added to some brands of breakfast cereals and other foods, but we don't have any idea what's still missing. Don't settle for "fortified" foods. You can be sure you are getting all the nutrients your body needs to process carbohydrates and stay healthy, by eating your carbohydrates the way nature intended – IN fruits, vegetables, whole grains and beans.

HOW REFINED CARBOHYDRATES CAN HARM YOU

All refined sugars and most refined grain products (anything made from flour, milled corn or white rice) have had vitamins, minerals and other nutrients removed in processing. Some but not all of these nutrients may be added back in enriched flours or fortified foods.

From 1600 to 1930, more North Americans died from the vitamin deficiency diseases, beriberi and pellagra, than from any other cause. These diseases disappeared when governments legislated that all flour had to have three vitamins, thiamin, niacin and riboflavin left in or added back. Over the last 70 years, the incidence of heart attacks in the United States had been increasing until Congress legislated that folic acid must be left in or added back to flour; now the heart attack rate is decreasing. However, diabetes and obesity continue to increase at alarming rates in all age groups.

Where carbohydrates are found in plants, the B vitamins are also found. Carbohydrates are combinations of sugars, either as single sugars or chains of sugars from two to millions. When you eat carbohydrates, enzymes in your intestines break them down into single sugars and only single sugars can pass from your intestines into your bloodstream, where they can be used for energy, stored as sugar in your liver or muscles or be converted to fat. Many different chemical reactions then break down sugar one step at a time to release energy. Each reaction must be started by an individual chemical called an enzyme and the B vitamins are parts of these enzymes that start the reactions that break sugar into energy.

If any of the B vitamins are not available, the conversion of carbohydrates to energy is blocked. Instead, the carbohydrates are converted to into fat which:

- raise blood levels of triglycerides;

- uses up the good HDL cholesterol, which lowers blood levels of HDL and increases risk for heart attacks;

- is stored in fat cells primarily in your abdomen;

- helps form plaques in arteries, which makes them stiff and raises blood pressure; and

- blocks insulin receptors on cells so you cannot respond adequately to insulin. This causes you to produce more insulin, which makes you hungrier, makes you store more fat, and leads to diabetes in susceptible people.

When you eat carbohydrates that have been separated from the B vitamins, minerals and perhaps other nutrients which have not yet been identified, you increase your risk for diabetes, obesity, heart attacks and high blood pressure. We do not have enough dependable research to know if taking the B vitamins separately (in other foods or supplements) is as healthful as eating the B vitamins as they come in nature, paired directly with the carbohydrates in whole grains and other seeds, vegetables and fruits.

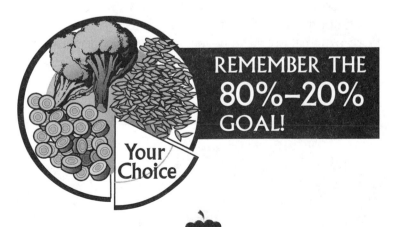

FIBER

Fiber is the structural material of plants and is found in all fruits, vegetables, whole grains, beans, nuts and other seeds. It is a type of carbohydrate that your body cannot break down, so you can't absorb it. There are two types: soluble and insoluble. Insoluble fiber adds bulk to your stool and helps to prevent constipation. Soluble fiber binds to fat in the intestines and keep some fat from being absorbed.

Insoluble fiber may help to prevent colon cancer by speeding cancer-causing agents through the digestive system. It helps with weight control because it binds to water, creating bulk that makes you feel full. It can help to control diabetes because it slows the rate at which your body absorbs glucose.

Soluble fiber has an added benefit. When you add more soluble fiber to your diet, it lowers blood levels of the plaque-forming LDL cholesterol. Soluble fiber is degraded by bacteria in the colon to form types of fatty acids that are absorbed into the bloodstream and help to block the synthesis of cholesterol by the liver. This is the only food component we know will lower blood cholesterol when you add more to your diet. However, people who have high blood levels of cholesterol must do a lot more than just add soluble fiber to their diet. They also should not smoke, not be overweight, and exercise regularly.

You should eat at least 35 grams of fiber per day, and the average North American gets only 11 grams. There's very little fiber in the typical diet of hamburgers, pizza, fried chicken and coke. Foods made from animal products never have any fiber, and processed foods made from grains, vegetables or fruit frequently have most of the fiber removed. Wheat berries, baked potatoes, apples and oranges contain many times more fiber than bread, potato chips, apple jelly or orange juice.

Don't worry about whether you are getting soluble or insoluble fiber; you need both kinds, and both are found in fruits, vegetables, whole grains and beans. If you're not getting enough fiber, don't try to correct the situation by adding fiber supplements, bran cereals or foods made with added ground-up fiber. When you eat whole fruits, vegetables, whole grains and beans, you get all of the vitamins, minerals and phytochemicals nature packages with the fiber. Introduce more high-fiber whole foods into your diet gradually to avoid digestive discomfort.

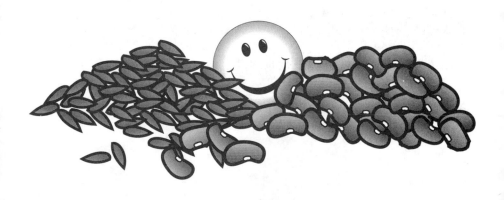

VITAMINS

Vitamins are chemical compounds which the human body needs to grow and function normally. Of the eleven vitamins we know humans need, nine are abundant in plants. Your body makes vitamin D from sunshine (or you can eat it in milk, eggs and fish). Vitamin B12 is found only in animals, and is often added to plant based foods such as cereals or soy milk.

Most of the vitamins humans need are synthesized by plants, so you get plenty when you eat a variety of fruit, vegetables, whole grains, beans and other seeds.

The B vitamins (thiamin, riboflavin, niacin, pyridoxine, folate, cyanocobalamin and biotin) are needed to convert carbohydrates into energy and for hundreds of other functions. They are found in whole grains, beans and many other plants, and in the animals that eat these plants.

Vitamins A, C and E are called the antioxidant vitamins because one of their important jobs is to prevent certain oxidizing chemical reactions that can be harmful to your body. The antioxidant vitamins help to prevent heart disease because LDL cholesterol must be oxidized before it can form plaques in your arteries. Brightly colored fruits and vegetables are particularly good sources of the antioxidant vitamins.

You can get all the vitamins you need from the food you eat. A daily multi-vitamin for extra "insurance" won't hurt you, but an unhealthy diet with vitamin pills is an unhealthy diet. Don't be tempted to try mega-doses of vitamins or high-priced supplements that make extravagant promises. You'll be wasting your money and can cause problems when you take too much of some vitamins.

MINERALS

Most of the minerals we need are the same ones plants require for their own growth. We both need: carbon, hydrogen, oxygen, nitrogen, phosphorous, potassium, sulfur, calcium, magnesium, iron, boron, manganese, copper, zinc, molybdenum and chlorine.

Plants don't store minerals just for our benefit — they use them for their own life cycles. If any of their 16 essential elements is not available, the plant withers and dies. If you buy a tomato or a red bell pepper, you know that the plant grew successfully and had all of the minerals it needed. If you eat a wide variety of foods from plants, you will get plenty of all these minerals.

The minerals we need that plants don't need are sodium, iodine, fluoride, selenium and cobalt. They may be in plants, but the plants don't die if they're not available. Most people get plenty of these minerals because our diet is abundant in salt, our water is fluoridated, and we eat foods grown in many different locations. Plants grown far from the oceans lack iodine, and a person who ate only those plants would have goiter, but this condition is no longer seen in North America because we use iodized salt and eat foods from all parts of the continent.

If you eat a moderately varied diet, you should get all the minerals you need and your body regulates them efficiently. Strict vegetarians should check the amount of calcium in the foods they eat, and may wish to take supplements or foods fortified with calcium.

PHYTOCHEMICALS

Plants contain hundreds of other chemicals that are useful to humans in addition to vitamins and minerals. These substances are grouped under the name *phytochemicals* (phyto=plant, chemical=chemical). The functions of some phytochemicals have been identified, but there are probably hundreds, or even thousands, that we have not yet discovered or do not understand their use to humans.

The plants we eat today are survivors of 3.5 billion years of competition. In the "survival of the fittest", the successful plants have developed a wide array of defenses against bacteria, fungi, wounds, insects and foraging animals. Humans have also evolved to benefit from some of these substances; these are the phytochemicals.

Our ancestors also learned to avoid plants that are poisonous to humans. Substances in edible plants that are harmless or beneficial in small quantities can be toxic in large amounts, so you should never eat huge amounts of any one plant, even if it contains beneficial substances. When you hear that a new phytochemical has been identified, don't rush out and eat huge amounts of that fruit or vegetable, or buy a pill that contains the new substance. Just continue to eat a wide variety of the fruits, vegetables, whole grains, beans and seeds and you'll benefit from ALL of the phytochemicals.

3. HOW TO USE THE FOOD LISTS

Most diet and nutrition books list all the foods you should avoid. This is a list of all the good foods you can choose from – foods that are full of the nutrients you need to stay healthy and help to prevent diseases. Remember the 80%—20% goal: if 80% of the foods you eat are on this list, and you select a wide variety, you'll have a healthy diet. You can do whatever you like with the other 20%.

The general goals of healthy eating apply to everyone, but you may have some special circumstances. See the suggestions in Chapter 5 if you have:

- Diabetes
- Heart problems or high cholesterol
- High blood pressure, or you
- Need to lose weight

The symbols ☺ 🥕 🥜 will guide you with choices to fit your special situation. Here's what they mean:

🥕 These are nutrient-rich foods that contain sugars or starches that cause blood sugar to rise quickly, which is a concern for diabetics and people who need to lose weight. They include fruits, root vegetables, and whole-grain products made with flour such as whole wheat bread, whole grain pastas and breakfast cereals. If you are diabetic or trying to lose weight, eat fruits and root vegetables only as part of a meal, so the other foods eaten at the same time will slow the release of sugars into your bloodstream. Try to avoid the products made with ground-up grains as much as possible, using whole grains (the seeds themselves) instead. See page 100.

These are nutrient-rich foods that are also concentrated sources of calories. They include nuts and snack seeds, seafood and dairy products. People who want to lose weight, lower cholesterol or control high blood pressure need to control the portion size of these foods because they can add a lot of calories without filling you up. Unless you are a strict vegetarian, we recommend 2-3 servings of skim milk dairy products each day and 4-6 ounce servings of seafood 2-3 times a week. With nuts and snack seeds, a reasonable serving size is 1-2 tablespoons per day. See page 59.

These nutrient-rich vegetables, whole grains and beans are bulky and have lots of fiber, so they fill you up; it would be very difficult to eat too much. Most people can eat as much of these foods as they like, as often as they like. Make them the centerpiece of your meals.

*Note: If your doctor has given you special diet instructions, please follow them regardless of the information contained in this book. If you have questions about what is appropriate for you, consult your doctor or health care provider.

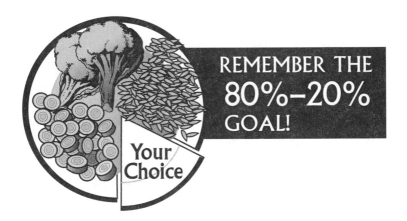

REMEMBER THE
80%–20%
GOAL!

Your Choice

4. FOOD LISTS

VEGETABLES

Vegetables come from all parts of the plant kingdom. We consider grains, beans, fruits and nuts as separate categories of foods, and lump all of the other edible parts of plants as "vegetables." This catch-all food group includes leaves (lettuce, spinach, kale); stalks (celery, asparagus), flowers (artichokes, broccoli, cauliflower), young seeds (green peas, lima beans) and roots or tubers (carrots, beets, potatoes.) Fruits that are not sweet, such as tomatoes, peppers and eggplants, are usually considered vegetables as well.

Most vegetables have a very high water content and lots of fiber, so they add a lot of bulk to meals without many calories. The colors of vegetables give clues to their vitamin content: darker green vegetables are usually good sources of B vitamins, while red and yellow ones are high in vitamins A and C; but all vegetables contain vitamins, minerals and phytochemicals, so everyone should eat as wide a variety as possible.

The nutritional content of vegetables is usually highest in those that are eaten fresh-picked and raw, but not always. Some phytochemicals are not released until the vegetable is cooked; for example, tomato sauce and tomato paste are better sources of lycopene than fresh tomatoes. The nutrient content of frozen and canned vegetables is plenty high enough to make them worthwhile additions to your meals. Variety is the key; eat the widest possible array of raw and cooked vegetables, selected and prepared to suit your tastes, your budget and your convenience.

 Root vegetables: Some plants have storage roots or tubers that contain large amounts of starch or sugar. They include carrots, potatoes, beets, parsnips, sweet potatoes, yams, yuca, taro and various tropical roots.

Root vegetables should be treated with the same caution as fruits by people who are diabetic or trying to lose weight: eat them in combination with other foods, not by themselves. A baked potato or carrots eaten by themselves as snacks will cause a sharp rise in blood sugar, but if you avoid them completely, you deprive yourself of their vitamins and phytochemicals. When you eat them with other foods, you slow the rise in blood sugar. (Watery, fibrous root vegetables such as radishes or onions do not require this caution.)

VEGETABLES, FRESH

- ☺ Alfalfa sprouts
- ☺ Amaranth leaves
- ☺ Arugula
- ☺ Artichokes
- ☺ Asparagus
- 🥜 Avocados
- ☺ Bamboo shoots
- ☺ Bean sprouts
- ☺ Beans, green
- ☺ Beans, yellow snap
- ☺ Beans, lima
- ☺ Beet greens

- ☺ Bok choy
- ☺ Broccolli
- ☺ Broccoflower
- ☺ Broccolini
- ☺ Brussels sprouts
- ☺ Cabbage
- ☺ Cabbage, Chinese
- ☺ Cabbage, Napa
- ☺ Cabbage, red
- ☺ Cabbage, savoy
- ☺ Cauliflower
- ☺ Celery
- ☺ Chard, swiss
- ☺ Chayote
- ☺ Collards
- ☺ Corn
- ☺ Cress, garden
- ☺ Cucumbers
- ☺ Dandelion greens
- ☺ Eggplant
- ☺ Endive
- ☺ Escarole
- ☺ Fennel

- ☺ Grape leaves
- ☺ Kohlrabi
- ☺ Leeks
- ☺ Lettuce
- ☺ Mizuni greens
- ☺ Mushrooms
- ☺ Mustard greens
- ☺ Okra
- ☺ Onions
- ☺ Onions, spring or green
- ☺ Palm hearts
- ☺ Peas, black-eyed
- ☺ Peas, green
- ☺ Peas, snow
- ☺ Peas, sugar snap
- ☺ Peppers
- ☺ Pumpkin
- ☺ Radicchio
- ☺ Radishes
- ☺ Rapini
- ☺ Seaweed
- ☺ Shallots
- ☺ Soybeans, green

☺ Spinach

☺ Squash, summer

☺ Squash, yellow

☺ Squash, crookneck

☺ Squash, zucchini

☺ Squash, winter

☺ Squash, butternut

☺ Squash, acorn

☺ Squash, hubbard

☺ Squash, spaghetti

☺ Swiss chard

☺ Tomatillos

☺ Tomatoes

☺ Water chestnuts

☺ Watercress

☺ All other vegetables
except root vegetables

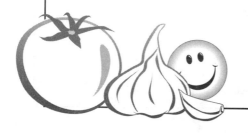

VEGETABLES, FROZEN

- ☺ Artichokes
- ☺ Asparagus
- ☺ Beans, green
- ☺ Beans, yellow snap
- ☺ Beans, lima
- ☺ Beet greens
- ☺ Broccolli
- ☺ Brussels sprouts
- ☺ Cauliflower
- ☺ Chard, swiss
- ☺ Collards
- ☺ Corn
- ☺ Mustard greens
- ☺ Okra
- ☺ Onions
- ☺ Peas, black-eyed
- ☺ Peas, green
- ☺ Peas, snow
- ☺ Peppers
- ☺ Soybeans, green
- ☺ Spinach
- ☺ Squash, summer

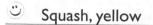 Squash, yellow

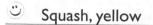 Squash, zucchini

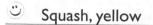 Frozen mixed vegetables

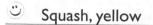 All other frozen vegetables except root vegetables

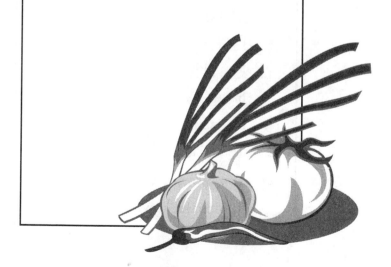

VEGETABLES, CANNED

☺ Artichokes

☺ Asparagus

☺ Bamboo shoots

☺ Beans, green

☺ Beans, yellow snap

☺ Beans, lima

☺ Collards

☺ Corn

☺ Grape leaves

☺ Mushrooms

☺ Mustard greens

☺ Okra

☺ Palm hearts

☺ Peas, black-eyed

☺ Peas, green

☺ Peppers

☺ Pumpkin

☺ Sauerkraut

☺ Spinach

☺ Tomatoes

☺ Tomatoes, crushed

☺ Tomatoes, stewed

☺ Tomato sauce

☺ Tomato paste

☺ Tomato puree

☺ Water chestnuts

☺ Vegetable soups

☺ All other canned vegetables except root vegetables

VEGETABLES, DRIED

☺ Mushrooms, dried

☺ Seaweed, dried

☺ Vegetable soup mixes

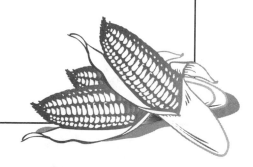

ROOT VEGETABLES, FRESH

- Beets
- Carrots
- Celeraic, celery root
- Jerusalem artichokes
- Jicama
- Parsnips
- Potatoes
- Rutabagas
- Saisify
- Sweet potatoes
- Taro
- Turnips
- Yuca
- Yams
- All other root vegetables

ROOT VEGETABLES, FROZEN

- Beets
- Carrots
- Potatoes
- Sweet potatoes

ROOT VEGETABLES, CANNED

- Beets
- Carrots
- Potatoes
- Sweet potatoes

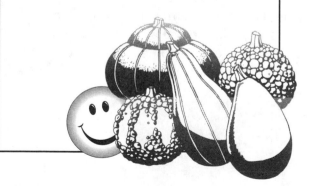

FRUITS

Fruits are the parts of plants that hold the seeds. Many plants rely on animals to carry seeds away from the parent plant, and have evolved with a wide array of ways to attract their helpers. Bright colors, tantalizing aromas and flavors appeal to humans as well as to many other species of mammals, birds and insects.

Fruits are loaded with vitamins, minerals and phytochemicals. Fruits are bulky foods, with lots of fiber and water so they are filling without contributing a lot of calories.

Fresh, raw fruits usually have the highest nutritional value, but frozen, canned and dried fruits retain plenty of their nutrients as well. Just choose as wide a variety as possible and eat several servings of fruits every day. Eat the peel if it's edible; vitamins, minerals and other nutrients are often concentrated in or near the skin.

Take advantage of the wide variety of fruits available in virtually every market; don't limit yourself to just apples, oranges and bananas. Count the number of different kinds of fruit you eat this week, then try to eat twice as many different ones next week.

Most fruits contain a lot of sugar, but that does not mean they should be avoided by diabetics or others who are concerned about sugar intake. No one should miss out on all the nutrients found in fruits; just eat them with other foods to avoid the rise in blood sugar that occurs in some individuals if fruit is eaten all by itself.

FRUITS, FRESH

- Apples
- Apricots
- Asian Pears
- Bananas
- Blackberries
- Blueberries
- Cactus Pears
- Carambola (Star Fruit)
- Cherimoyas
- Cherries
- Clementines
- Coconut
- Cranberries
- Currants
- Dates
- Feijoa
- Figs
- Gooseberries
- Grapefruit
- Grapes
- Guavas
- Kiwi fruit

- Kumquats
- Lemons
- Limes
- Lychees
- Mangoes
- Melons
- Nectarines
- Oranges
- Papayas
- Peaches
- Pears
- Persimmons
- Pineapple
- Plantains
- Plums
- Pomegranates
- Pomelos
- Prunes
- Pumpkin
- Quinces
- Raisins
- Raspberries
- Rhubarb

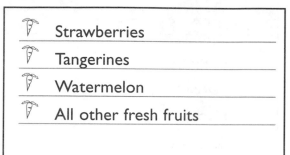

| Strawberries |
| Tangerines |
| Watermelon |
| All other fresh fruits |

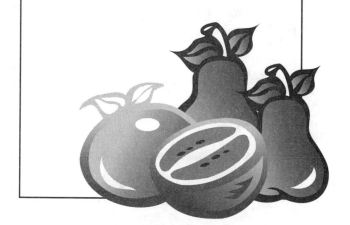

FRUITS, FROZEN

🥕 Apples

🥕 Apricots

🥕 Blackberries

🥕 Blueberries

🥕 Cherries

🥕 Mangoes

🥕 Melons

🥕 Nectarines

🥕 Oranges

🥕 Papayas

🥕 Peaches

🥕 Raspberries

🥕 Rhubarb

🥕 Strawberries

🥕 Mixed frozen fruits

🥕 All other frozen fruits

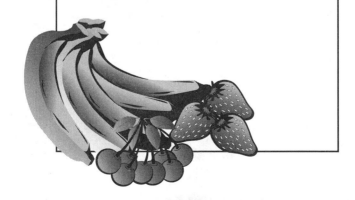

FRUITS, CANNED

- Apples
- Apricots
- Blackberries
- Cherries
- Cranberries
- Grapefruit
- Lychees
- Peaches
- Pears
- Pineapple
- Plums
- Prunes
- Pumpkin
- Raspberries
- Rhubarb
- Mixed canned fruits
- All other canned fruits

FRUITS, DRIED

- Apples
- Apricots
- Bananas
- Blueberries
- Cherries
- Coconut
- Cranberries
- Currants
- Dates
- Figs
- Mangoes
- Papayas
- Peaches
- Pears
- Pineapple
- Plantains
- Prunes
- Raisins
- Raspberries
- Strawberries
- Mixed dried fruits
- All other dried fruits

WHOLE GRAINS

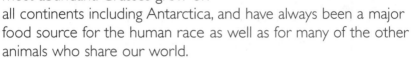

W hole grains are the seeds of grasses. The grass family is one of the largest plant families on our planet (more than 10,000 kinds) and one of the most abundant. Grasses grow on all continents including Antarctica, and have always been a major food source for the human race as well as for many of the other animals who share our world.

Whole grains were the first food humans learned to cultivate, marking our transition from hunter-gatherers to agricultural societies. The various grasses that grew in different parts of the world — rice, corn, wheat, rye, oats, quinoa, amaranth, teff, millet — became the "staff of life" for ancient societies. Our ancestors relied heavily on grains because they are easy to grow and store; and they are excellent food, providing lots of carbohydrates for energy plus protein, fat, vitamins and minerals.

Today we have dozens of varieties of whole grains, and a huge array of whole-grain products to choose from. There are so many choices that you don't ever need to eat foods made from refined grains (white flour, white rice or milled corn) that have had valuable nutrients and fiber removed. If you are trying to lose weight or are diabetic, try to use actual whole grains (whole seeds such as brown rice, wild rice or barley) as often as possible. These are marked with the ☺ symbol. See Chapter 6 for more information on whole grains.

WHOLE GRAINS

☺ Amaranth

☺ Barley

☺ Buckwheat groats

☺ Corn, dried

☺ Kamut

☺ Kasha, whole (buckwheat)

☺ Kashi (mixed grains)

☺ Millet

☺ Oat groats

☺ Popcorn (air popped)

☺ Quinoa

☺ Rice, black, Japonica

☺ Rice, brown, basmati

☺ Rice, brown, jasmine

☺ Rice, brown, long grain

☺ Rice, brown, medium grain

☺ Rice, brown, short grain

☺ Rice, brown, other varieties

☺ Rice, wild & brown mix

☺ Rye Berries

☺ Spelt

☺ Teff

☺ Triticale

☺ Wheat berries, all varieties

☺ Wheat berries, sprouted

☺ Wild rice

☺ Any other whole grains (seeds)

WHOLE GRAIN PRODUCTS

🌱 Bulgur

🌱 Couscous, whole wheat

🌱 Oats, rolled

🌱 Oats, steel-cut

🌱 Wheat, cracked

🌱 Wheat germ

🌱 Whole grain pastas

🌱 Whole grain breads (see page 46)

🌱 Whole grain cereals (see page 48)

🌱 Other whole grain products

Diabetics and people who are trying to lose weight or control cholesterol should avoid all forms of ground-up grains, and that includes bread. For everyone else, bread is a perfectly satisfactory food.

Breads have been made for thousands of years, in virtually every culture, to wrap, sandwich, or accompany other foods for breakfast, lunch and dinner. When ground-up grains were used shortly after milling, there was no need to remove anything or to add ingredients to keep them fresh. Only in our recent history have we turned bread into junk food by removing the germ and fiber from the grains. Even worse, some bread manufacturers add partially hydrogenated fats to their breads to prolong their shelf life.

The best way to assure that you are getting a bread that is made from whole grains, with nothing removed, is to bake your own bread made from flour you grind yourself, or buy from local bakers who grind their flour fresh every few days (these are hard to find.) Not many people are going to be able to do that. So here are my goals for picking the best of the commercial breads:

1. Avoid any bread that is made with partially hydrogenated oils. Read the list of ingredients and if it contains the words partially hydrogenated, put it back on the shelf. Partially hydrogenated oils are totally unnecessary for making good-tasting bread, and we should boycott the companies that use them in their products until they get rid of them. The prime offenders are Pepperidge Farm, Arnold and Brownberry brands.

2. Get as much whole grain flour as possible. This isn't easy to tell, because regulations allow bread makers to use the words whole wheat even if portions of the grain have been removed. Words like stone ground, multi-grain, seven-grain or cracked wheat sound healthy but don't tell you anything. Generally, breads that list whole wheat as the first ingredient are better than those that start with enriched flour of some sort.

3. Pick breads with higher fiber content. 2 grams of fiber per slice is better than 1 or 0 grams. One caution: breads promoted for their fiber content may have added pea fiber or some such ingredient; that's adding sawdust, not an indication that you're getting the whole grains. Check the list of ingredients on these breads.

4. Added seeds are a bonus. Many breads include seeds in the dough or as toppings. This is an easy way to add caraway seeds, sesame seeds, poppy seeds or other whole seeds to your diet.

5. Breads made from 100% sprouted grains have all the nutrients of whole grains, may have more vitamins, and may raise blood sugar less than breads made with dry flour.

6. Watch out for breads that taste too good. Nothing is more seductive than a loaf of freshly baked bread. A reasonable portion is 1-2 slices. If you eat the whole loaf in one sitting, or the whole basket of rolls in a restaurant before dinner comes, you'll get into trouble.

HOW TO PICK A BREAKFAST CEREAL

The healthiest breakfast is whole grain cereal. If you're trying to lose weight, control cholesterol or diabetes, or just need a lot of energy, your best bet is a hot cooked cereal of whole grains, such as oat groats, barley or wheat berries, served like oatmeal - perhaps with cinnamon or raisins. Most of the prepared hot cereals such as oatmeal are made from whole grains and are just fine, too, but not as filling.

If you prefer cold cereal, you need to check the list of ingredients carefully. The FIRST ingredient should be a whole grain. Then scan through the entire list and if you see the words "partially hydrogenated," put the box back on the shelf. You should avoid foods with partially hydrogenated oils (or "trans fats"), and they show up in an alarming number of cereal brands

Once you've eliminated all the brands made with refined grains or partially hydrogenated oils, check for added sugars (you want little or none) and fiber (you want a lot.)

The fiber content listed on the nutrition label can be confusing because it's based on serving size, and very light cereals (such as puffed wheat) show little fiber per serving, but an acceptable amount when you adjust for weight. Cereals made from bran (the outer covering removed from whole grains) will have higher fiber content than cereals made from whole grains (which have the germ and starchy parts of the grains as well as the fiber), but they can be hard to digest.

BREAKFAST CEREALS, WHOLE GRAIN

- Cheerios—General Mills
- Chex, Wheat—General Mills
- Grape Nuts—Post
- Healthy Choice Toasted Brown Sugar Squares—Kelloggs
- Just Right with Fruit & Nuts—Kelloggs
- Mini-Wheats, Raisin Squares—Kelloggs
- Mini-Wheats, Frosted, Bite-Size—Kelloggs
- Mini-Wheats, Frosted—Kelloggs
- Muesli—Familia
- Nutri-Grain, Golden Wheat—Kelloggs
- Nutri-Grain, Almond-Raisin—Kelloggs
- Oatmeal Crisp, Almond—General Mills
- Oatmeal Crisp, Apple Cinnamon—General Mills

- Oatmeal Crisp, Raisin—General Mills
- Oatmeal Squares—Quaker
- Organic Healthy Fiber Multigrain Flakes—Health Valley
- Puffed Wheat—Quaker
- Shredded Wheat—Post
- Shredded Wheat & Bran—Post
- Shredded Wheat, Frosted—Post
- Shredded Wheat, Spoon Size—Post
- Total, Whole Grain—General Mills
- Wheaties, Crispy 'n' Raisins—General Mills

BREAKFAST CEREALS, HIGH-BRAN

🌱 100% Bran—Post

🌱 All Bran, bran buds—Kelloggs

🌱 All-Bran, extra fiber—Kelloggs

🌱 All-Bran, original—Kelloggs

🌱 Bran Flakes—Post

🌱 Chex, Multi-Bran—General Mills

🌱 Complete Wheat Bran Flakes—Kelloggs

🌱 Complete Oat Bran Flakes—Kelloggs

🌱 Fiber 7 Flakes—Health Valley

🌱 Fiber One—General Mills

🌱 Oat Bran—Quaker

🌱 Oat Bran Flakes—Health Valley

🌱 Oat Bran Flakes with Raisins—Health Valley

🌱 Organic Bran with Raisins—Health Valley

🥕 Raisin Bran—Kelloggs

🥕 Raisin Bran Flakes—Health Valley

🥕 Raisin Bran, Whole Grain Wheat— Post

🥕 Total, Raisin Bran—General Mills

BEANS AND OTHER LEGUMES

Legumes are our second most-important food source (grains rank first). Humans consume huge amounts of both beans and grains, and use even more to feed livestock we raise for meat, dairy products and eggs.

The huge legume family includes the many varieties of beans, as well as lentils, peas and peanuts. Here we are concerned with the dry seeds of legumes that have been staples in our diet for thousands of years. (Fresh beans and peas are grouped with Vegetables, page 25, while products made from soybeans have their own section, page 61.) Beans, like grains, are easy to grow and store so they were among the first plants to be cultivated when humans moved from hunting-gathering to agriculture.

Seeds contain everything necessary to bring a new plant to life, so they are nutritional powerhouses for us as well. They provide vitamins, minerals and phytochemicals; and are very high in fiber. They are good sources of essential fatty acids and are the best plant source of protein. While most beans do not contain all of the essential amino acids (see page 12), eating them with grains yields "complete" protein. Our ancestors figured this out, since virtually every culture has devised tasty combinations of beans and grains that have provided sustinance for generations. Many of our favorite recipes today are based on these traditional dishes.

Most supermarkets carry a wide variety of dried and canned beans. They are equally nutritious. Dried beans are usually more economical, but they take longer to prepare. Canned beans are more convenient; it's your choice. Canned "baked beans" may contain added sugar and fat, so check the list of ingredients if this is a concern for you.

Beans come in lots of colors and sizes, and there are different popular names for some varieties. For example, chick peas are also called garbanzo beans or chana dal. All beans are cooked basically the same way and their flavors are similar., so they are usually interchangeable in recipes. Pick your favorite kinds or use whatever is available.

Most legumes are relatively low in fat, with most of their energy (calories) coming from protein and carbohydrates. However, soybeans, peanuts and some of their relatives are concentrated sources of fat and need to be treated with caution by those who are trying to control their weight or cholesterol.

BEANS, DRIED

☺ Adzuki beans

☺ Appaloosa beans

☺ Black beans

☺ Blackeyed peas

☺ Broad beans

☺ Butter beans

☺ Cannellini

☺ Chick peas

☺ Chili beans

☺ Cranberry beans

☺ Fava beans

☺ Flageolets

- ☺ Garbanzo beans
- ☺ Great Northern beans
- ☺ Haricot beans
- ☺ Kidney beans
- ☺ Lentils, brown
- ☺ Lentils, French green
- ☺ Lentils, orange
- ☺ Lima beans, baby
- ☺ Lima beans, large
- ☺ Mung beans
- ☺ Navy beans
- ☺ Peanuts
- ☺ Peas, whole dried
- ☺ Pigeon peas
- ☺ Pink beans
- ☺ Pinto beans
- ☺ Rattlesnake beans
- ☺ Red beans
- ☺ Roman beans
- 🫘 Soy beans
- ☺ Split peas, green
- ☺ Split peas, yellow

☺	White beans, small
☺	Mixed beans
☺	Bean soup mixes
☺	Bean soup cups
☺	All other dried beans

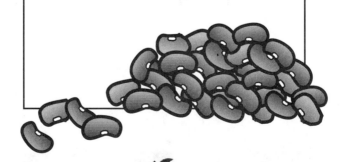

BEANS, CANNED

☺ Adzuki beans

☺ Baked beans, vegetarian

☺ Black beans

☺ Blackeyed peas

☺ Broad beans

☺ Butter beans

☺ Cannellini

☺ Chick peas

☺ Chili, vegetarian

☺ Fava beans

☺ Flageolets

☺ Garbanzo beans

☺ Great Northern beans

☺ Kidney beans

☺ Lentils

☺ Lima beans, baby

☺ Lima beans, large

☺ Mung beans

☺ Navy beans

☺ Pigeon peas

☺ Pink beans

🙂	Pinto beans
🙂	Red beans
🥜	Soy beans
🙂	White beans, small
🙂	Bean soups
🙂	All other canned beans

NUTS AND SNACK SEEDS

All seeds are highly nutritious packages containing protein, minerals, vitamins, fiber and phytochemicals, plus a calorie source for the baby plant — fat, carbohydrates or both. The oil seeds, such as nuts, olives, corn, cottonseed, peanuts, flaxseeds and soybeans have a large percentage of fat, and it's mostly "good" fats — polyunsaturated and monounsaturated fats. Their polyunsaturated fats include varying amounts of the essential fatty acids (omega-3's and omega-6's).

A reasonable daily amount of any of these seeds is 1-3 tablespoons. That's why we caution you to watch out for nuts if you're trying to lose weight. It's practically impossible for the most rational human to stop at a tablespoon of salted peanuts or almonds. Each tablespoonful is about 100 calories. A 12.5-ounce can of peanuts is 2200 calories. It's easier to just avoid temptation. It's much easier to limit the portion size of seeds used for flavoring, such as sesame, poppy, caraway, cumin or fennel; or those that have virtually no flavor, such as flax seed.

Salted nuts ARE an ideal food to take along for prolonged, intense exercise like cycling or running: They're easy to carry, concentrated energy, and the salt plus the fluid you drink with them keep you from getting dehydrated.

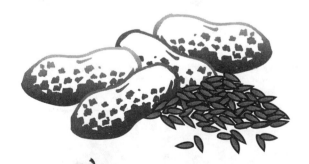

NUTS AND SNACK SEEDS

- Almonds
- Brazil nuts
- Cashew nuts
- Chestnuts
- Coconut
- Filberts
- Flax seeds
- Hazelnuts
- Macadamia nuts
- Peanuts
- Pecans
- Pine nuts, pinons, pignolas
- Pistachios
- Pumpkin seeds
- Sunflower seeds
- Walnuts
- Mixed nuts
- All other nuts & snack seeds

SOY PRODUCTS AND
VEGETARIAN MEAT SUBSTITUTES

Most larger supermarkets carry a variety of soy products, including veggie burgers, ground meat substitutes, tofu and soy milk. Vegetarian burgers come in a huge array of flavors and brands; they can be prepared quickly in a microwave and served with the condiments you'd use on a conventional burger. The ground soy "meats", found either in the produce section or the frozen food section, can be used any way you would use ground beef.

Soy milk is labeled "soy beverage" and is usually not displayed in the dairy section; you may need to ask where your store keeps it. It's ideal for people who are lactose-intolerant as well as for vegetarians. It doesn't curdle when heated.

All dried beans and the foods made from them are good sources of protein, fiber, vitamins and minerals. Soybeans have the added attraction of phytoestrogens, and they are a good source of omega-3 fatty acids. A diet that includes soy products may reduce the symptoms of PMS and menopause, and may help to prevent certain cancers. However, too much soy, like any other excess, is unwise.

The U.S. Food and Drug Administration recently approved special health claims for soybean products. Unfortunately, this may lead some people to eat unreasonably large amounts of soybean products. If you eat a lot of any one food, you may harm yourself, even though reasonable amounts are harmless or beneficial.

SOY PRODUCTS AND OTHER VEGETARIAN FOODS

- Soybeans
- Soy nuts, roasted
- Soy grits
- Soy sprouts
- Soybeans, green (edamame)
- Texturized Vegetable Protein (TVP)
- Tofu
- Soymilk
- Soy cheese
- Soy yogurt
- Okara
- Tempeh
- Mochi
- Miso
- Soy burger
- Soy Canadian bacon
- Soy ham
- Soy pepperoni

- Soy sausage
- Soy turkey
- Soy hotdogs
- Seitan
- Vegetable burgers
- Almond milk
- Oat milk
- Multi-grain milk
- Rice milk
- Other soy products

SEAFOOD

Seafood is a good source of protein, minerals, vitamins and essential omega-3 fatty acids. Fish contain more polyunsaturated fats and less saturated fats than meats from animals that are raised on land (beef, pork, poultry, lamb.) However, you can get all of the nutrients found in fish from other sources, so vegetarians are not missing anything essential if they avoid seafood.

The richest sources of omega-3's in seafood are the fatty fish that live in cold, deep water. Tuna, salmon, swordfish, sardines, herring, mackerel and anchovies are examples of deep-water fish. Clams, crab, squid, shrimp and other seafood also contain omega-3's.

One easy way to increase the amount of omega-3 fats in your diet is to eat canned fish two or three times a week. Water-packed tuna or salmon can be added to salads or eaten just as they come from the can. Sardines packed in mustard sauce or tomato sauce make tasty snacks.

The amount of fat in tuna varies from fish to fish, and the canner must measure and label each batch to reflect the actual fat content. That's why you may find two cans of the exact same brand and style of water-packed tuna, one with 1 gram of fat per serving and another with 5 grams per serving. This is one time that more fat is better; the fattiest tuna contains the most omega-3's.

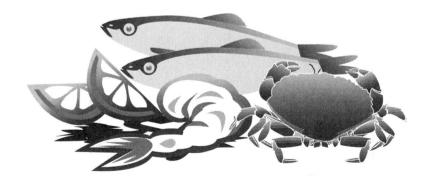

While some fish have little fat and others have quite a lot, they all have the 🥜 symbol in the lists. That's because they have no fiber, so they are not very filling. Limit your portion size if you need to control diabetes, cholesterol or high blood pressure, or are trying to lose weight. A reasonable serving is 3-4 ounces.

High concentrations of heavy metals have raised concerns about the safety of some seafoods, so we recommend that you not eat large amounts of a single type of fish caught in any one location. This is one more reason to eat a varied diet and not to eat too much of any one food. We also recommend that you avoid raw seafood; some fish contain parasites that are harmful to humans, but they are killed by cooking.

SEAFOOD

🥜 Albacore

🥜 Amberjack

🥜 Anchovies

🥜 Bass

🥜 Bass, sea

🥜 Blackfish

🥜 Bluefish

🥜 Bonito

🥜 Butter fish

🥜 Carp

🥜 Catfish

- Clams
- Cod
- Conch
- Crab, Alaska
- Crab, blue
- Crab, Dungeness
- Crab, king
- Crab, snow
- Crab, softshell
- Crabmeat, imitation
- Crawfish or crayfish
- Croaker
- Dolphin
- Drum
- Eel
- Flounder
- Grouper
- Haddock
- Hake
- Halibut
- Hoki
- Herring

- Langostino
- Lobster, American
- Lobster, Spiny
- Mackerel
- Mahi-mahi
- Marlin
- Monkfish
- Mullet
- Mussels
- Octopus
- Orange roughy
- Oysters
- Perch, Lake
- Perch, Ocean
- Petrale
- Pike
- Pike, walleye
- Pollock
- Pompano
- Porgy
- Redfish
- Red snapper

- Rockfish
- Salmon
- Sand dabs
- Sardines
- Scallops, bay
- Scallops, sea
- Shad
- Shark
- Sheepshead
- Shrimp
- Shrimp, rock
- Skate
- Smelts
- Snails
- Snapper
- Sole
- Squid
- Sturgeon
- Surimi
- Swordfish
- Tautog
- Tilapia

- Tilefish
- Trout, brook
- Trout, lake
- Trout, rainbow
- Trout, sea
- Tuna
- Turbot
- Walleye
- Weakfish
- Whitebait
- Whitefish
- Whiting
- Yellowtail
- All other seafood

DAIRY PRODUCTS

Skim milk and skim milk products such as yogurt and cottage cheese are good sources of protein, calcium, vitamin D and other nutrients. Unless you are a strict vegetarian or are lactose intolerant, it makes sense to include 2-3 servings of skim milk dairy products each day. Whole milk, cheese and other full-fat dairy products are high in saturated fats so are best limited by everyone except for young children and high-performance athletes who burn huge amounts of calories.

People who are lactose-intolerant or vegan have plenty of other choices; most supermarkets now carry an array of soy beverages and other plant-based milk substitutes such as rice milk or almond milk. Use the nutrition labels on these products to guide your selection, since they vary widely in the amounts of calcium, vitamin B12 and nutrients they contain.

While skim milk dairy products have little or no fat, they all have the 🍪 symbol in the lists. That's because they have no fiber, so they are not very filling. Limit your portion size if you need to control diabetes, cholesterol or high blood pressure, or are trying to lose weight. A reasonable serving is one cup of milk or yogurt, or 1-2 ounces of cheese.

Don't let advertising campaigns persuade you to drink huge amounts of milk. Several studies that show that osteoporosis is associated far more with taking in too much protein, than with not getting enough calcium in the diet. Taking in too much protein causes the body to convert protein building blocks called amino acids into organic acids that acidify the blood. The kidneys respond by neutralizing the blood by taking calcium from bones and pushing it out through the urine. Two or three cups of milk is reasonable; six or eight cups a day is not.

DAIRY AND EGG PRODUCTS, NON-FAT

- Milk, non-fat
- Milk, lactose-free, non-fat
- Yogurt, non-fat, plain
- Cottage cheese, non-fat
- Evaportated milk, non-fat
- Egg whites
- Egg substitutes, non-fat
- Other fat-free dairy products

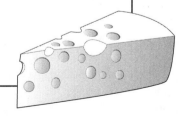

HERBS, SPICES AND SEASONINGS

Most whole grains, vegetables and beans have bland flavors that would be boring without herbs, spices or other seasonings. Spices are usually seeds, used whole or ground. Some spices are roots, bark or other plant parts, either fresh (as in ginger root) or dried (as in cinnamon bark.) Herbs and spices contain a variety of vitamins, minerals and phytochemicals, but they are usually used in such small amounts that they do not make a significant contribution of either calories or other nutrients to your diet.

While any leafy green may be called an herb, we usually reserve this word for the leafy parts of highly-flavored plants that are used for seasoning. Their assertive flavors and aromas add interest and distinction to recipes of different cultures. You can grow your own fresh herbs or buy them in supermarkets or ethnic markets; dried herbs are widely available.

Many traditional seasonings are made from combinations of spices and other ingredients: prepared mustard, horseradish, Worcestershire sauce and many other condiments provide special flavors and convenience. As with spices and seasonings, their flavors are usually strong and distinctive, so only small amounts are needed to add interest to recipes or at the table.

HERBS, FRESH

- 😊 Basil
- 😊 Chervil
- 😊 Chives
- 😊 Cilantro, coriander, Chinese parsley
- 😊 Dill weed
- 😊 Fennel
- 😊 Garlic
- 😊 Ginger root
- 😊 Lemon grass
- 😊 Marjoram
- 😊 Mint
- 😊 Oregano
- 😊 Parsley
- 😊 Parsley, Italian or flat
- 😊 Rosemary
- 😊 Sage
- 😊 Tarragon
- 😊 Thyme
- 😊 All other fresh herbs

HERBS AND SPICES, DRIED WHOLE OR GROUND

☺ Allspice

☺ Anise

☺ Apple pie spice mix

☺ Basil

☺ Bay leaves

☺ Bouquet garni

☺ Cajun spice mix

☺ Cayenne pepper

☺ Caraway seeds

☺ Cardamom

☺ Celery seeds

☺ Chervil

☺ Chili powder

☺ Chinese five spice mix

☺ Chives

☺ Cilantro

☺ Cinnamon

☺ Cloves

☺ Coriander seeds

☺ Cumin seeds

- ☺ Curry powder
- ☺ Dill seeds
- ☺ Fennel seeds
- ☺ Fennugreek seeds
- ☺ Garam masala mix
- ☺ Garlic
- ☺ Ginger
- ☺ Mace
- ☺ Marjoram
- ☺ Mustard, dried
- ☺ Mustard seeds
- ☺ Nutmeg
- ☺ Oregano
- ☺ Paprika
- ☺ Parsley
- ☺ Pepper, black
- ☺ Pepper, red
- ☺ Pepper, white
- ☺ Pepper, cayenne
- ☺ Pickling spices
- ☺ Poppy seeds
- ☺ Pumpkin pie spice mix

☺	Saffron
☺	Sage
☺	Sesame seeds
☺	Thyme
☺	Tumeric
☺	Vanilla beans
☺	Spice mixes
☺	All other spices

SEASONINGS AND CONDIMENTS, PREPARED

☺ Anchovy paste

☺ Bean dip

☺ Black bean sauce, Asian

☺ Bouillon cubes, granules, paste, liquid

☺ Catsup

☺ Curry pastes

☺ Fish sauce, Asian

☺ Ginger, pickled

☺ Hoisin sauce

☺ Horseradish

☺ Hot pepper sauces

☺ Liquid smoke seasoning

☺ Mustard, prepared

☺ Olives

☺ Oyster sauce

☺ Pickles, unsweetened

☺ Salsa

☺ Steak sauces

☺ Tabasco sauce

☺ Vanilla extract

☺ Vinegar

☺ Wasabi

☺ Worcestershire sauce

☺ Other seasoning sauces and condiments

5. SPECIAL SITUATIONS

DIABETICS

EAT LOTS	CAUTION

CAUTION

— Eat fruits and root vegetables only with meals.

— Avoid bread and other foods made from flour or ground-up grains as much as possible – use whole grains instead.

— Limit if you need to lose weight.

All diabetics should eat lots of fruits, vegetables, whole grains, beans and other seeds, and deep water fish. They should restrict meat, chicken, whole milk dairy products, bakery products, pastas, all sugar added products and all food with partially hydrogenated fats. Fruits and root vegetables should be eaten only with other foods.

Soon after you eat, your blood sugar level rises. If it rises above the normal of 160, sugar sticks to cells membranes and it can never detach. It is converted to a poison called sorbitol that damages the cells to cause all the side effects of diabetes such as blindness, deafness, burning foot syndrome, heart attacks, strokes or kidney damage.

Diabetes is treated by keeping blood sugar levels from rising too high after meals. A diabetic should avoid refined carbohydrates such as bakery products, pastas, sugar-added products and fruit juices. They should also avoid saturated fats and partially hydrogenated fats, which bind to insulin receptors and prevent your body from responding to insulin, causing blood sugar levels rise too high.

Most diabetics also need to lose weight, and fats are the most concentrated sources of calories. Meat, chicken and whole milk dairy products are high in saturated fat, and partially hydrogenated fats are found in many packaged foods, fried foods, fast foods and solid margarines, so diabetics should avoid these foods as well as the refined carbohydrates.

Many diabetics need medication to get their diabetes under control, but you may be able to get off all medication once you lose weight and make a permanent change in your eating habits. For information on the most effective medications, the latest research and tips for getting diabetes under control, visit the Diabetes section of www.drmirkin.com. See also the tips for losing weight on pages 82-83.

HEART PROBLEMS, HIGH CHOLESTEROL & HIGH BLOOD PRESSURE

EAT LOTS

CAUTION

— If overweight, eat fruits and root vegetables only with meals.

— Avoid bread and other foods made flour or ground-up grains as much as possible — use whole grains instead.

— Limit if you need to lose weight.

For the last 60 years, doctors have told us that a high-fat diet causes heart attacks. Now a study from Harvard Medical School shows that eating lots of refined carbohydrates can also cause heart attacks.

The glycemic index measures how high a person's blood sugar rises after eating a certain food in comparison to blood sugar rise with sugar. A study of 75,000 women showed that those most likely to suffer a heart attack ate the most foods that cause the highest rise in blood sugar. High glycemic index foods include all those that have added sugar such as pastries, cakes, cookies and most soft drinks; those made from flour such as bakery products and pastas; fruit juices; root vegetables such as potatoes and beets; and fruits.

A diet rich in fruits and vegetables and low in fat is far more effective in lowering high blood pressure than a low-salt diet.

Now, preventing heart attacks must include not only reducing your intake of added fats, particularly saturated and partially hydrogenated fats; you should also avoid refined carbohydrates. Eat lots of vegetables, whole grains, beans, seeds and nuts. People who are also overweight or diabetic should eat fruits and root vegetables only in combination with other foods to slow the rise in blood sugar.

OVERWEIGHT

EAT LOTS

CAUTION

— Eat fruits and vegetables only with meals.

— Avoid bread and other foods made from flour or ground-up grains as much as possible — use whole grains instead.

— Limit serving sizes.

The only ways to lose weight (without surgery or prescription medications) are:

1. *Take in fewer calories,* **2.** *Burn more calories, or* **3.** *both.*

All of the popular diet books, regardless of the "scientific" explanations they give, recommend menus that give you 1500-1800 calories or less per day, and for most people this means you will be taking in fewer calories. You can lose weight on any low-calorie diet, but ask yourself: Is this a way of eating I can follow for the rest of my life? (If not, you will regain the weight as soon as you go back to your old eating habits.) And, do the foods they tell me to eat supply all the nutrients my body needs? Most people can eliminate whole food groups for a short time without any harm, but eventually you will create deficiencies if you do not eat a wide variety of foods, with lots of fruits, vegetables, whole grains, beans and other seeds. Don't believe that you can make up for what's missing with pills: a lousy diet with supplements is a lousy diet.

The sensible way to lose weight is to eliminate the foods with little or no nutritional value beyond the concentrated calories they contain: refined carbohydrates and added fats. The guidelines for diabetics (page 79) apply for anyone who needs to lose weight, particularly if you store most of your weight in your belly. Avoid foods that raise insulin to high levels such as bakery products, pasta, and foods with added sugars. You should eat enough whole grains, beans, and vegetables to keep you full and satisfied. Eat root vegetables and fruits only with other foods.

It's better to eat several small meals than one or two large ones. After you eat, your body temperature rises to burn extra calories because food must first be broken down by multiple chemical reactions that produce a lot of heat. If you eat only one large meal, you produce extra heat for only a few hours. When you nibble small amounts more often, you produce extra heat throughout the day and burn far more calories.

The Fitness section of www.drmirkin.com has lots of ideas to help you start and maintain an exercise program. The latest research on weight loss and healthy eating are reported in the Nutrition section.

When one person in a household needs to lose weight, the whole family needs to cooperate. Foods made with refined carbohydrates and added fats should be kept out of the house. Everyone will benefit from eating more vegetables, whole grains and beans.

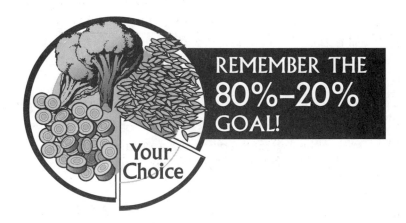

REMEMBER THE
80%–20%
GOAL!

Your Choice

CHILDREN
EAT LOTS

Children learn about food best by seeing the adults around them eat in a healthy way. Meals should not be a battleground. Keep junk out of the house, offer lots of choices from all the foods in this book, and don't make an issue over food likes and dislikes.

You can involve your children in food preparation and meal planning with activities that are appropriate for their age. This can provide opportunities to learn about food and experiment with new tastes. Keep it fun and sociable.

If weight is a concern, increase physical activity. Large children may be athletically gifted and should be encouraged to participate in sports and do weight training. As with food choices, the example set by parents and other adults will be more important than anything you say. Get active as a family. Hike, bike or swim together. Don't make children feel they should limit the amount of food they eat – just steer them away from "junk" food as much as possible. Kids will eat anything and everything outside the house, so you can only influence what's available at home.

There are no easy solutions to the alarming increase in childhood obesity, type II diabetes and early puberty, but you can make a start by limiting refined carbohydrates in your house, serving lots of fruits, vegetables, whole grains, beans and other seeds, and getting the whole family involved in active recreation.

SENIORS
EAT LOTS

Just as you may lose the sharpness of your vision or hearing with age, seniors may find that their senses of taste and smell are less sharp than they once were. Seniors often lose interest in food just because it doesn't taste as good as it once did. Try more spices and seasonings, bold flavors and new tastes and textures to keep food interesting.

Work on staying active, or becoming more active so you can continue to eat a wide variety of nutritious foods as you age without consuming too many calories.

It's never too late to begin an exercise program. Underweight older people look and feel frail because they have lost most of their muscles, not because of lack of fat. If you are inactive, you lose muscle mass to the point where you are unable to carry out daily activities — climbing stairs, getting up out of a chair — because your muscles are not strong enough to move the weight of your own body. Don't try to add fat to a weak body.

Overweight older people often have the double burden of weak muscles AND 20, 40 or more extra pounds to lug around with them every day. See page 82

ATHLETES & ACTIVE TEENS
EAT LOTS

   plus whatever else you need to meet your calorie requirements.

It takes a lot of energy to power your muscles for an athletic competition. Your brain gets its energy almost exclusively from sugar in your bloodstream and your muscles don't contract effectively when your blood sugar runs low. There is only enough sugar in your bloodstream to last three minutes, so to keep sugar levels from dropping, your liver releases sugar from its cells. But your liver stores only enough sugar to last 12 hours. Eating fills your liver with sugar. If you eat six hours before you compete, your liver will already have used up a major portion of its stored sugar, so you want to fill your liver with sugar as close to your event as possible and leave your stomach empty. That's two to three hours before competition. You don't need to eat sugar; your body converts any type food you eat to sugar for energy.

Protein helps your muscles recover faster after a hard workout. Weight lifters and other athletes often use protein supplements or special protein drinks, but they are no better than the protein found in food. Just eat a big meal with dairy products, fish, beans or other high-protein foods after your workout or game.

Athletes in training and active teens involved in sports may burn as many as 7500 calories a day. It's hard to eat that much food. You should eat huge amounts of the foods listed here to get the vitamins, minerals and phytochemicals your body needs, plus anything else — ice cream, cheese, pizza, steaks, chocolate bars, whatever you like. Remember, saturated fats and refined carbohydrates only cause problems when they are not burned for energy. People who burn 7500 calories a day need to eat everything in sight.

PREGNANT OR NURSING
EAT LOTS

The latest research show that pregnant women should eat lots of nuts, seeds, whole grains, beans, fruits and vegetables; restrict added vegetable oils and and avoid all packaged foods that contain partially hydrogenated fats.

Both mother and child need essential fatty acids that are classified into omega-3s and omega-6s. Pregnancy uses up fatty acids, particularly omega-3s such as docosahexaenoic acid (DHA). Several recent studies show that post-partum depression is caused by low levels of omega-3 fatty acids. Essential fatty acids are found in all nuts, seeds, beans and whole grains, but not in refined flour used for most bakery products and pastas. Seafood is also a good source of omega-3's.

Pregnancy depletes folic acid, and a deficiency can cause birth defects. Folic acid is found in leafy greens, nuts, seeds and beans. Extracted oils from seeds such as corn, soybeans, cottonseed, rapeseed (canola) and safflower are often converted to partially hydrogenated fats and added to foods. These fats deplete the body of omega-3 fatty acids and therefore should be avoided by pregnant women.

WANT TO GAIN WEIGHT
EAT LOTS

If you think you're too thin and want to gain weight, don't just sit on the couch and stuff yourself with food. Weight gain should always be in the form of muscle, not fat. To build muscle, start a weight-bearing exercise program. Go to a gym and learn how to do the weight training circuit. Build up those arms and legs! As you exercise, your appetite will respond to meet your needs. It only takes 15 extra grams of protein a day to build a pound of muscle a week — so you really won't need to eat a lot more. Muscle weighs more than fat.

Once you are exercising regularly and gaining muscle, your appetite will probably increase and you will eat more without any conscious effort. Most muscular people and heavy exercisers will eat plenty to meet their calorie needs. The training tables for football teams are piled high with every kind of food.

Don't worry if you lose weight because of a temporary illness. You will recover your appetite and return to your normal weight, gradually, without overeating. However, unexplained weight loss is a serious concern and should be reported to your doctor.

MUST EAT IN RESTAURANTS OFTEN
EAT LOTS

LIMIT (FOR MANY PEOPLE)

Everyone can enjoy an occasional meal in a restaurant and order whatever they want. But if you have to eat in restaurants several times a week, you need to devise ways to make healthy choices and avoid the temptation to over-eat. If you are trying to control weight, diabetes, cholesterol or high blood pressure, you need to must find ways to meet your special requirements.

First, choose restaurants that gives you a fighting chance. Find a restaurant with a good salad bar and load up on fresh vegetables. Order broiled fish for your entree. Ask to have it prepared with lemon juice instead of butter. Have steamed vegetables as an accompaniment, without added butter, and fresh fruit or fruit ice for dessert.

Asian restaurants often have a wide array of tasty dishes with lots of vegetables. Thai and Vietnamese restaurants and Mongolian grills are good choices if you stick to the vegetarian and seafood entrees. Go easy on the white rice.

Your chances of finding whole grains in a restaurant are slim to none, but if you travel a lot, you might want to pack or shop for your own cereal to eat in your hotel. Large cities and college towns often have vegetarian restaurants that offer varied, flavorful meals made with vegetables, beans and sometimes even whole grains.

Whatever you order, watch out for the huge portions that many restaurants serve. Divide it up at the beginning of the meal and save some for the next day's lunch, share with a friend, or just leave it.

The restaurants listed below are a few of the national chains that offer good to excellent salad bars and some other healthier choices for people on the go.

Black Eyed Pea

Bob's Big Boy

Chili's

Denny's

Golden Corral

Long John Silvers

Lone Star

Olive Garden

Ponderosa

Ruby Tuesday

TGI Friday's

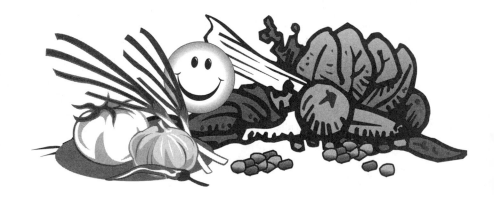

JUST TOO BUSY FOR HEALTHY EATING?
EAT LOTS

Everyone is busy! Here are a few easy ways to add more healthy foods to your hectic days.

1. Find a whole grain cereal that tastes good dry, and use it for snacking or breakfast on the run. See the list of recommended cereals (pages 48-50).

2. Make your own fast food. Once a week, cook up a huge pot of chili, soup, or one of my vegetable or seafood casseroles. Freeze the leftovers in individual serving containers for quick suppers or lunches.

3. Cook a pound of whole grains at a time, and freeze the left-overs in 1/2 to 1-cup portions in baggies. These can be reheat-ed in the microwave in seconds. Chapter 6.

4. Stock up on the dried soup cups that have beans or lentils as their main ingredient. Find flavors you like and use them for lunch at the office or on the run — anywhere you can get hot water. Mix with one of those baggies of whole grains for a hearty main dish.

5. Find a few veggies that you like raw and unadorned to eat as you would eat fruit. Try red bell peppers, green beans and cau-liflower.

6. Romaine hearts, packed in plastic bags, can be used as-is for quick salad preparation. Just tear or slice into bite-size pieces. Good even without dressing.

7. Most Asian restaurants offer carry-out service. This is a good standby for lazy days. Vietnamese restaurants often have wonderful, oil-free salads that keep for 2-3 days. Comb the menu for soups, vegetable and seafood dishes and ask them to go easy on the oil. Serve them with those whole grains from their baggies in your freezer!

8. Large grocery stores and specialty food stores often have salad bars and prepared food sections. You need to be careful about your choices, but if you are strong-willed (and not too hungry when you shop), you can usually find plenty of vegetables, fruits, and possibly some seafood entrees among their offerings.

9. Take advantage of pre-cut vegetables and fruits in your supermarket's produce department, and bags of mixed vegetables in the frozen food section. The time you save can make up for the added cost.

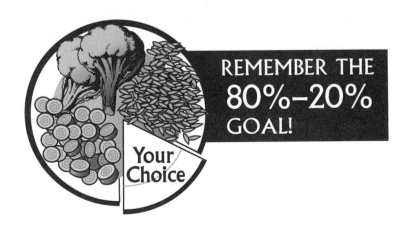

REMEMBER THE
80%–20%
GOAL!

Your Choice

6. USING WHOLE GRAINS

Once you decide to add whole grains in your diet, you will find that you have lots of choices. Some of the names may seem confusing at first, but most of the whole grains are interchangeable in recipes. All of the whole grains have bland, neutral flavors and can be used any way you would use pasta or white rice. You can add them to soups, top them with your favorite chili or pasta sauce, or use them to make hearty salads. They are also delicious as hot breakfast cereals or in rice-pudding type desserts. Many of the recipes in the next section call for cooked whole grains. Follow the directions in this chapter and keep a variety of cooked whole grains on hand in your freezer, ready to make your own healthy "fast food."

WHERE TO FIND WHOLE GRAINS

Most larger supermarkets carry wild rice, barley and brown rice. They may all be in the section with white rice and pasta, or you may find barley in the international section (with Jewish specialties) and wild rice in the gourmet food section. Your supermarket may have a health section with various other whole grains (the selection varies widely from store to store and region to region.) You will probably need to go beyond your supermarket to find some of the less common whole grains such as kamut or oat groats. Try the health food stores, specialty gourmet shops, and food co-ops in your area. Or you can order whole grains by mail at www.gethealthyshop.com or call (800)420-4726.

HOW TO STORE WHOLE GRAINS

Uncooked whole grains keep a long time in canisters or other air-tight containers. If you plan to store grains for several months, use containers made of glass, metal or hard plastic to avoid insects. They will keep even longer if you store them in your refrigerator or freezer.

Cooked whole grains should be refrigerated and will keep about a week in a covered container. If you don't plan to use them up in a few days, put leftovers in portion-size freezer containers or plastic sandwich bags and freeze them. They are ready to serve after a minute or two in the microwave.

HOW TO COOK WHOLE GRAINS

Ignore the instructions on packages of whole grains — use the charts on the next pages instead. You do not need to rinse or pre-soak whole grains. The first time you cook a new grain, check them 5-10 minutes before the end of the cooking time to make sure they are not getting mushy. If they aren't tender enough to suit you at the end of the recommended time, cook a little longer.

Cook grains in bouillon or other flavored liquid. You can use bouillon cubes, granules, liquid or paste; make up the required amount of liquid following the directions on your brand of bouillon. Grains cooked in vegetable or chicken flavored bouillon will have a neutral flavor that can be used for any purpose: breakfast cereal, main dishes, salads or desserts. If your bouillon does not contain salt, add a little salt to your taste. Whole grains cooked without any salt will taste flat.

COOKING WHOLE GRAINS IN A STEAMER

If you are serious about healthy eating, get an electric countertop steamer. This is by far the easiest, most convenient way to cook all of the whole grains. Look for one with at least an 8-cup capacity rice bucket and 75-minute timer. Countertop steamers come with instruction booklets with detailed information for cooking vegetables and seafood. Follow these instructions for cooking whole grains, using the times and amounts shown in the chart.

Fill the steamer base with water to the top line. (Do not use the drip tray.) Place the steamer basket on the base. Place the grains and bouillon (use amounts from the chart) in the rice bowl and set the rice bowl in the steamer basket. Cover, plug in, and set the timer. Let the grains sit for at least 20-30 minutes after the timer rings before removing the lid. You can let them sit for several hours if you prefer. This way you can let them cook while you sleep or go to work. Drain the grains in a colander if there is excess liquid.

FOR 21/2 CUPS (1 LB.) GRAINS:	AMOUNT OF BOUILLON	COOKING TIME
Wheat Berries	4 cups	75 minutes
Kamut	4 cups	75 minutes
Spelt	4 cups	75 minutes
Rye	4 cups	75 minutes
Triticale	4 cups	75 minutes
Oat Groats	4 cups	75 minutes
Barley	4 cups	75 minutes
Brown Rice	4 cups	65-75 minutes
Wild Rice (1/2 lb.)	4 cups	75 minutes
Millet	4 cups	40 minutes
Quinoa	4 cups	30 minutes
Amaranth	4 cups	30 minutes
Kasha (Buckwheat Groats)	4 cups	15-20 minutes

COOKING WHOLE GRAINS ON THE STOVETOP

Any of the whole grains can be cooked in a pot just as you would cook white rice, but they take longer and will use more liquid. Use a medium-size pot with a tight-fitting lid. Bring the liquid to a boil in the pot, stir in the grains and return to boiling. Reduce the heat to low, cover the pot and simmer until the grains are tender and most of the water is absorbed. Drain off any excess liquid.

FOR 2 1/2 CUPS (1 LB.) GRAINS:	AMOUNT OF BOUILLON	COOKING TIME
Wheat Berries	6 cups	60 minutes
Kamut	6 cups	60 minutes
Spelt	6 cups	60 minutes
Rye	6 cups	60 minutes
Triticale	6 cups	60 minutes
Oat Groats	6 cups	60 minutes
Barley	6 cups	60 minutes
Brown Rice	5 cups	45 minutes
Wild Rice (1/2 lb.)	6 cups	60 minutes
Millet	5 cups	20 minutes
Quinoa	5 cups	15 minutes
Amaranth	5 cups	20 minutes
Kasha (Buckwheat Groats)	6 cups	15 minutes

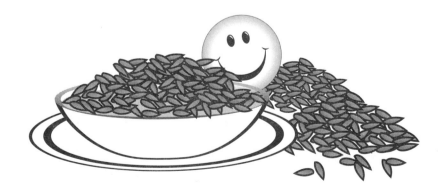

OTHER COOKING METHODS

You can add raw grains to soups or stews while they cook, but it may be hard to get everything done at the same time without overcooking any of the ingredients. Some of the recipes in this book use this method, but most recommend cooking the grains separately. Do whatever seems easiest for you.

Other appliances can be used to cook whole grains; try what you have on hand.

RICE COOKER

If you have a rice cooker with a metal container and no timer, you may be able to use it to cook your whole grains, but you will need to experiment. These cookers use a sensor to determine when the liquid has been absorbed. Start with the quantities listed on the steamer chart, page 95, and add more liquid if your grains come out too hard, less if they are too soft.

CROCKPOT

Put the quantity of grains and liquid listed on the stovetop chart into your crockpot or slow cooker, turn it on and leave it for 6-8 hours.

PRESSURE COOKER

If you're comfortable using a pressure cooker, they work just fine for whole grains. Follow the stovetop cooking chart and adjust the cooking times as you would for any other food (usually about half the regular time.)

A SIMPLE WAY TO COOK WHOLE GRAINS

The Fiber-Magic Whole Grain Cooker™ provides you with a quick and easy way to cook one to two cups of whole grains. It's a thermos-like container with a special heating material in the base. You put 1/2 cup of grains into the cooker, add water to the fill line, and microwave it uncovered for three minutes. Seal the cooker with its lid and shake. Then let it sit for two to three hours while the grains cook. You can take the cooker along with you to work or while you travel. Full instructions come with the cooker. The Fiber-Magic Cooker is available at www.gethealthyshop.com, or call (800)420-4726.

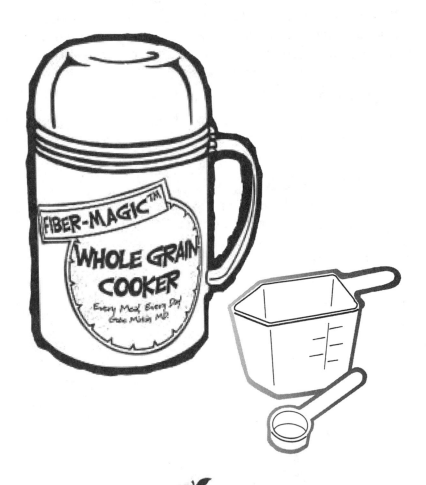

ANATOMY OF A GRAIN

When you eat whole grains, you are eating viable seeds — you can sprout them if you wish. All of the components of the seed are intact. As shown in the diagram, each grain or seed has four parts:

THE HUSK OR HULL is a papery outer covering that is always removed. Many grains fall out of their husks when they are harvested. A few grains (such as barley and buckwheat) have very hard hulls; these must be ground away. Grains that have the husk or hull removed are considered whole grains (and will still sprout) if the bran layers and the germ are intact.

BRAN LAYERS: Each seed is protected by an outer coating that is several layers thick. The bran layers are rich in fiber, vitamins and minerals.

GERM OR EMBRYO: This is the part of the seed that becomes a new plant if it is allowed to sprout. The tiny germ contains protein, essential fatty acids, vitamins and minerals. If the seed is broken open, the germ begins to turn rancid almost immediately, so it is usually removed when grains are ground into flour.

ENDOSPERM: The largest part of the seed feeds the growing embryo if it is allowed to sprout. It is virtually all starchy carbohydrates. The calorie-rich endosperm is what we eat when grains are refined to remove the coarse outer covering (the fiber) and the nutrient-rich but quick-spoiling germ.

Endosperm

Bran Layers

Germ

Husk

WHOLE GRAINS ARE BETTER THAN ANY FLOUR

When grains are processed into flour or cereals, the primary concern is loss of nutrients. However, if you grind your own grains or use products that are made from the whole grain without discarding anything, you get all or most of the nutrients of the original grain. But grains that have been broken apart in any way will be digested quicker. That's a big disadvantage for diabetics and dieters.

Carbohydrates are long chains of sugars, and only single sugars can be absorbed from your intestines into your bloodstream. The foods that cause rapid rise in blood sugar are those that are digested most quickly; the worst offenders are sugar and anything made from flour. When you eat whole grains (seeds), it takes a long time to break apart the capsule, separate the carbohydrates from the fiber, and completely digest each grain. Your blood sugar rises slowly, stays slightly elevated for a long time (so you don't feel hungry again soon after eating) and never reaches the high levels that come from sugar or flour.

Grains that are eaten as whole seeds are also more filling and satisfying because they have more bulk and take longer to break down. Part of their bulk comes from water: each seed swells up when it cooks and soaks up water, which is carried in the grain until it is completely broken down in your digestive tract. (The water you drink, on the other hand, is absorbed directly from your stomach almost as soon as it gets there. Water and other liquids do not "fill you up.") Processed grains absorb some water when you cook them, but less than the whole seeds; and the water is separated out more quickly during the digestive process. Most people can easily eat two or three cups of pasta, but you will find that you feel full with just a cup of whole grains, or even less.

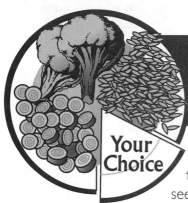

Your Choice

The whole grains are chewy and take more time to eat. Some of the seeds are broken apart by your chewing, but not all of them. Some of the grains may even pass through your system undigested. On the other hand, anything made from flour or grains that have been cut, flaked, rolled or shredded has been thoroughly pre-chewed and pre-digested for you. You may get all the nutrients of the whole grains, but you don't get the full benefits of bulk and slow transit through your digestive system.

Whole grain pastas, breads and cereals are certainly better than refined grain products, but to get ALL the benefits of whole grains, eat the seeds themselves

7. RECIPES

It's hard to go wrong when you cook with fruits, vegetables, whole grains and beans. You don't need to worry about precise measurements, cooking times or ingredient preparation. The recipes give you general guidelines, but if you do things a little differently, chances are your dish will still be delicious.

MEASUREMENTS: Most cooks don't do a lot of measuring. Recipes have to give measurements to give you some idea what the author has in mind. Measure out a teaspoon of salt and pour it into your hand to see what it looks like; then learn to use your eyes to measure. Use your taste buds, too. Taste as you go and adjust the seasonings to suit yourself.

When a recipe calls for ingredients like an onion, a potato, an orange or a green pepper, use average-sized vegetables or fruits. If yours are very small or large, just make a good guess about how much you should use. If you like an ingredient, feel free to add more; if you're not crazy about it, add less or leave it out (see Substitutions below.)

CHOP, SLICE, DICE, MINCE: Lots of recipes for fruits and vegetables instruct you to cut the ingredients up. How you do it is up to you. A knife and chopping board are easy to use and clean, but if you want to use a food processor or other favorite cutting device, go right ahead. You may enjoy cutting things into tiny, uniform pieces, but it's not necessary for these recipes. Generally, when the recipe says chop or dice, it means 1/4" to 1/2" chunks; anything smaller than bite-size is fine. Slice usually means cutting the ingredient crosswise into about 1/4" pieces. Mince means the pieces should be really small — 1/8" or so. To mince garlic, you may want to use a garlic press.

PEEL OR NOT?

Vegetable and fruit skins are loaded with fiber, vitamins and minerals. Don't throw them away unless you have to. Use this "rule of thumb" — if you can put your thumbnail through the skin, leave it on. This eliminates the tough ones like winter squash and the thick ones like banana and orange peels. If you think peeling is important for the texture or appearance of a recipe, go ahead, but at least think about it before you automatically throw away valuable fiber and nutrients.

COOKING TIMES

Cooking times in recipes are approximate. Your taste testing is far more important than the clock. The ultimate test is "doneness." Check a carrot or a potato and see if it's tender. Cook a dish long enough to blend the flavors but not so long that it turns to mush.

SUBSTITUTIONS

All of these recipes can be used as springboards for new inventions. Be creative! You may want to make changes to use up ingredients you have on hand; you may not be able to find an ingredient in the store; or you may just prefer some other ingredient or seasoning. You may want to make notes on the substitutions you've tried and the results. Do be brave about trying things you"don't like"; new combinations and seasonings can change your mind.

WHOLE GRAINS ARE INTERCHANGEABLE. All whole grains have bland flavors that are very similar to one another. They do have subtle differences in flavor and texture, so you will probably like some more than others (taste is highly individual.) Try several of the different types and decide which ones you like best. Then feel free to use your favorites in any of the recipes.

BOUILLON

Many of the recipes list "bouillon" in the ingredients. Use your favorite brand of bouillon or experiment with new ones until you find some you like. You can use plain water and a little salt if you wish, but bouillon gives a flavor boost.

Bouillon comes in many forms: cubes, granules, pastes and liquid concentrates that are added to water, or canned bouillons and broths that are ready-to-use. Follow the package directions to make up the amount of bouillon called for in the recipe; usually you will add one cube or one teaspoon of the product for each cup of water. If a recipe specifies bouillon granules or bouillon cubes, add them to the pot without additional water.

Vegetable or chicken flavored bouillons have neutral flavors that go well with any whole grains, beans or vegetables. Whole grains cooked in vegetable or chicken bouillon can even be used in the recipes for desserts and as hot breakfast cereal. Stronger flavors, such as beef, ham or fish bouillons, can be used in hearty recipes such as chilies or soups. The recipes were tested with bouillon granules that contain salt, and you will find salt in most prepared bouillons. If you use a low-salt brand, adjust the seasonings to your own taste.

SPICE BLENDS

Spice blends such as curry powder, chili powder and Cajun spice blend are a great shortcut for the busy cook who wants maximum taste with minimum effort. Most supermarkets carry a variety of spice blends, or you can make your own using the recipes on the next pages. Use them to add infinite variety to your combinations of whole grains, vegetables and beans.

Look for "mild" curry powder or chili powder and add the degree of heat you want with a little cayenne pepper or hot sauce such as Tabasco. If you don't like one spice blend, try another brand; each manufacturer has its own formula.

AFRICAN BERBERE SPICE BLEND

3 tbs sweet paprika
2 tsp ground cumin
1 tsp cinnamon
1 tsp tumeric
1 tsp dry ginger
1 tsp ground coriander ·
1 tsp nutmeg, mace or allspice
1/2 tsp cloves
1/2 tsp cayenne, or to taste

Mix all ingredients. Store in an airtight container.

Yield: About 1/4 cup

GARAM MASALA SPICE BLEND

2 tbs freshly ground black or white pepper
2 tsp ground cumin
2 tsp ground coriander
2 tsp cinnamon
1 tsp cardamon
1 tsp nutmeg
1/2 tsp cloves

Mix all ingredients. Store in an airtight container.

Yield: About 1/4 cup

HARISSA SAUCE (HOT!)

A little harissa goes a long way! Stir in a tiny bit while you cook, or let each person mix a little into their own portion of any vegetable or bean dish. Be sure to caution anyone who is not familiar with Harissa.

2 tbs cayenne
1 tbs ground cumin
1 tsp ground caraway
1 clove garlic
1/2 t. salt
1/4 cup fat-free Italian salad dressing

Mix the dry spices in a small refrigerator container. Peel the garlic clove and press it through a garlic press into the dry spices. Add the salad dressing and mix well. Store covered in refrigerator (keeps indefinitely.) Very hot!

Yield: About 1/4 cup

DESSERT SPICE BLEND

Hot breakfast cereals and whole grain desserts can be made more delicious with a cinnamon-based spice blend. Find a good "Apple Pie Spice" or "Pumpkin Pie Spice" in your supermarket or make your own with this recipe.

3 tbs cinnamon
1 tbs nutmeg
1 tbs dry ginger
1 tsp cloves
1 tsp cardamon
1 tsp mace

Mix all ingredients. Store in an airtight container.

Yield: About 1/4 cup

MAIN DISHES

RED PEPPER STEW

1/2 cup red lentils
1/2 cup small white beans
2 onions, chopped
3 cups bouillon
6 medium or 4 large red bell peppers,
cut in 1/2" chunks
1 teaspoon oregano or marjoram
1/2 teaspoon thyme
pinch of cayenne, or to taste
1 cup white wine
3 tablespoons tomato paste
1/4 cup chopped Italian parsley
freshly ground black pepper to taste
cooked whole grains (optional)
plain yogurt for garnish (optional)

Soak the lentils and beans in water overnight. Drain and set aside.
Combine the onions and bouillon in a large pot. Bring to a boil,
reduce the heat and simmer, uncovered, while you chop the peppers (5-10 minutes). Add the peppers, spices, wine, tomato paste,
and the soaked lentils and beans. Return to boiling, reduce the heat
and simmer, covered, for about an hour or until the beans are tender. Stir occasionally and add more bouillon if needed. When ready
to serve, stir in the parsley and black pepper. Serve over whole
grains or as a soupy-stew, topped with a spoonful of yogurt if
desired.

4-6 servings

JAMAICAN GUMBO

2 onions, chopped
2 cups bouillon
3 sweet potatoes, cut in 1/2" dice
1 small head cabbage, cored and shredded
2 tablespoons minced fresh gingerroot
1-2 jalapeno chiles, seeded and minced, or to taste
1 28-ounce can Italian plum tomatoes, undrained, broken up
1 box frozen sliced okra, or 2 cups fresh, cut in 1/2" slices
1 cup pineapple tidbits (fresh or canned)
Juice of 1 lime
1/4 cup chopped cilantro or Italian parsley
Cooked whole grains of your choice

Cook the onions in 1/2 cup of the bouillon to soften, about 5 minutes. Add the remaining bouillon, sweet potatoes, gingerroot, chiles and tomatoes. Bring to a boil, reduce the heat and simmer, covered, about 10 minutes or until the sweet potatoes are just tender. Stir in the okra and cook 10-15 minutes, until the okra is tender. Stir in the pineapple, lime and cilantro or parsley. Serve over the whole grains.

6-8 servings

EASY SWEET AND SOUR PEPPERS

For the sauce:
1 tablespoon cornstarch
1/2 cup water
1 clove garlic, crushed in garlic press
1/4 cup catsup
1/4 cup soy sauce
1/4 cup cider vinegar
2 tablespoons brown sugar

For the vegetables:

1/2 cup bouillon
1 bag frozen pepper-onion stir-fry mix
1 cup frozen or canned (drained) shoepeg corn
1 8-ounce can sliced water chestnuts, drained
2 cups cooked barley or other whole grains of your choice

Make the sauce: Mix the cornstarch and 2 tablespoons of the water into a smooth paste. Combine with the remaining water and the other sauce ingredients.

Heat the bouillon to boiling in a pot and add the frozen vegetables; stir until thawed and heated through. Add the remaining vegetables and the sauce; heat through. Serve over the whole grains of your choice.

4 servings

POTATO GOULASH

2 pounds medium red potatoes, cut in half lengthwise, then cut in 1/4" slices
1 onion, chopped
2 cloves garlic, minced
2 tablespoons sweet paprika
1 teaspoon caraway seeds
1 teaspoon oregano
1 28-ounce can Italian plum tomatoes and their juice, broken up
2 teaspoons bouillon granules
2 cups cooked barley or other whole grain of your choice

Combine all ingredients except the grains in a large pot. Bring to a boil, reduce the heat and simmer, covered, 30-40 minutes or until the potatoes are tender. Stir occasionally and add water if needed. Serve over whole grains.

4-6 servings

PICADILLO

1 onion, chopped

1 green pepper, chopped

2 cups canned Italian plum tomatoes, undrained, broken up

2 bouillon cubes or 2 teaspoons bouillon granules

1 12-ounce package veggie burgers, broken into small pieces, or frozen soy burger crumbles

1/2 cup stuffed green olives, sliced

1/2 cup golden raisins

1 tart apple, coarsely grated or chopped fine

1 tablespoon mild chili powder

2 teaspoons dessert spice blend or cinnamon

generous pinch of cayenne pepper, to taste

2 tablespoons red wine vinegar

2 tablespoons slivered almonds or pine nuts

Cooked whole grains of your choice

Combine the onion, green pepper, tomatoes and bouillon granules in a large pot. Bring to a boil, reduce the heat and simmer 5-10 minutes. Stir in the remaining ingredients except the nuts. Return to boiling, reduce the heat and simmer 15-20 minutes. Stir in the nuts. Serve over whole grains.

4-6 servings

SPANISH RICE

Of the whole grains, I think barley is better than brown rice as a substi-tute for white rice in this traditional dish. You can use any whole grain you prefer; the texture varies, but the flavor will be delicious.

1 onion, chopped
1 red bell pepper, chopped
1 green bell pepper, chopped
1 clove garlic, minced
2 tablespoons tomato paste
1 cup bouillon
4 cups cooked barley or brown rice
1 6-ounce can diced green chiles
1/2 cup sliced pimento-stuffed olives (optional)
chopped cilantro for garnish (optional)

Combine the onion, peppers, garlic, tomato paste and bouillon in a pot. Bring to a boil, reduce the heat and simmer, covered, 5-10 minutes, or until the vegetables are softened. Stir in the barley and cook 5-10 minutes more to blend the flavors. Add the chiles and olives, if using; serve garnished with cilantro if desired.

4-6 servings

WINTER SQUASH-FRUIT CASSEROLE

2 pounds butternut squash or other winter squash
1 large onion, chopped
1 clove garlic, minced
4 cups bouillon
2 tablespoons tomato paste
2 teaspoons curry powder
1 teaspoon nutmeg
 pinch cayenne, or to taste
2 tart apples, cored and cut in 1/2" chunks
1/2 cup dried cranberries
1 cup cooked barley or other whole grain
  of your choice
ground cinnamon for garnish

Pierce the squash with a knife in 2
or 3 places. Set in a microwave dish
and microwave on high for 3 minutes or until it can be cut easily.
When cool enough to handle, cut the
squash in half and scoop out the seeds. Cut the squash
into bite-size pieces; peel or not, as you wish.

Meanwhile, combine the onion, garlic, bouillon, tomato paste, curry
powder, nutmeg and cayenne in a large pot. Bring to a boil, reduce
the heat and simmer 5-10 minutes. When the squash is ready, add it
to the pot and cook until the squash is barely tender, about 10 minutes. Add the apples, cranberries and the barley and cook 10-15
minutes more, until the apples are tender. Dust each serving with a
pinch of ground cinnamon if desired.

4-6 servings

GARDEN RISOTTO

1 cup baby carrots, cut in 1/4" slices
2 shallots, chopped
1 cup bouillon
pinch cayenne, or to taste
1/2 pound asparagus, cut in 1/2" pieces
1/2 cup frozen peas
1 small yellow squash, cut in 1/2" cubes
2 cups cooked oat groats, barley
   or other whole grain of your choice
2 cups slivered fresh spinach leaves (see note)
1/2 cup slivered fresh basil leaves (see note)

Note: to sliver the spinach and basil, take a handful of the leaves, roll them up and slice crosswise into thin shreds (1/8" - 1/4" wide)

Combine the carrots, shallots, bouillon and cayenne in a pot. Bring to a boil, reduce the heat and simmer, covered, about 5 minutes or until the carrots are just tender. Add the asparagus, peas and squash; return the liquid to a boil, then reduce the heat and simmer until the asparagus is just tender, 3-5 minutes more. Stir in the whole grains, spinach and basil and heat through.

4-6 servings

WILD RICE JAMBALAYA

1 pound shrimp
3 cups bouillon
1 bay leaf
1 tablespoon Cajun spice
1 onion, chopped
1 green pepper, chopped
3 stalks celery, chopped
2 cloves garlic, minced
2 cups canned Italian plum tomatoes,
   undrained, chopped
1 cup uncooked wild rice or rice blend
1 bunch green onions, chopped
1/4 cup chopped Italian parsley
Freshly ground black pepper
Tabasco Sauce (optional)

Peel the shrimp, reserving the shells. Set the shrimp aside. Add the
shrimp shells, bouillon, bay leaf and Cajun spice blend to the pot,
bring to a boil and simmer 10-15 minutes while chopping the vegetables. Strain the bouillon and return it to the pot; discard the
shrimp shells. Add the onion, green pepper, celery, garlic, tomatoes
and rice to the bouillon and simmer, covered, for 45 minutes, or
until the rice is tender. Stir in the shrimp, green onions and parsley
and cook 3-4 minutes, or until the shrimp is pink and firm. Serve
with ground pepper and Tabasco Sauce to taste.

6-8 servings

POLYNESIAN BEANS AND GRAINS

1 onion, chopped
1/2 cup bouillon
2 tablespoons hoisin sauce or oyster sauce
1 tablespoon soy sauce
1 tablespoon Dijon-style mustard
2 tablespoons tomato paste
1 teaspoon cumin
1 orange
1 cup fresh or canned pineapple chunks (reserve juice)
2 cans pink beans, drained
2 cups cooked whole grains of your choice

Combine the onion, bouillion and seasonings in a pot. Bring to a boil, reduce the heat and simmer, covered, 5-10 minutes. While the sauce is cooking, grate the rind of the orange into the pot.

Remove the remaining orange peel, section the orange and cut each section into bite-size pieces. Add the orange pieces, pineapple, beans and grains to the pot and heat through. If the mixture seems too dry, add a little of the pineapple juice.

4-6 servings

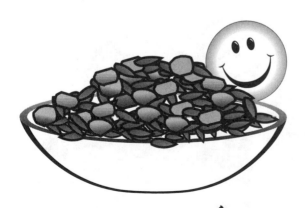

MENESTRA (SPANISH VEGETABLE STEW)

1 large onion, chopped
4 cloves garlic, minced
2 cups bouillon
2 carrots, sliced
2 medium red potatoes, cut in 1/2" chunks
2 tablespoons sweet paprika
2 bay leaves
pinch cayenne, or to taste
1/2 cup dry sherry
1 red bell pepper, cut in 1/2" chunks
1 8-ounce box mushrooms, quartered
1 14-ounce can artichokes, drained and cut in bite-size pieces
1 cup frozen peas
cooked whole grains of your choice

Combine the onion, garlic and bouillon in a large pot. Bring to a
boil, reduce the heat and simmer 5 minutes while preparing the
other vegetables. Add the carrots, potatoes , spices and sherry.
Return the liquid to boiling, then reduce the heat and simmer until
the vegetables are just tender. Add the bell pepper, mushrooms and
artichokes and simmer 5-10 minutes. Stir in the peas and serve over
the whole grains of your choice.

4-6 servings

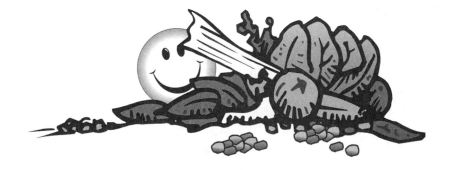

CABBAGE TAGINE

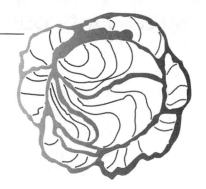

2 onions, halved lengthwise,
   then sliced thin

2 cups bouillon

1 tablespoon grated fresh gingerroot

2 teaspoons ground coriander

1/2 teaspoon tumeric

1/2 teaspoon cinnamon

pinch cayenne, to taste

1 small head cabbage, quartered,
   then sliced crosswise into 1/4" strips

1 red bell pepper, cut in 1/4" x 1" strips

2 cups canned Italian plum tomatoes, undrained, chopped

1 16-ounce can chick peas

1/4 cup dried cherries or raisins

2 tablespoons lemon juice

1/4 cup chopped cilantro (optional)

cooked whole grains of your choice

Combine the onions, bouillon and spices in a large pot. Bring to a
boil, reduce the heat and simmer while preparing the other vegetables. When the cabbage is ready, stir it in. Add the red bell pepper,
tomatoes, chick peas and cherries and simmer, uncovered, 10-15
minutes. Stir in the lemon juice, and the cilantro if desired, and
serve over the whole grains of your choice

4-6 servings

 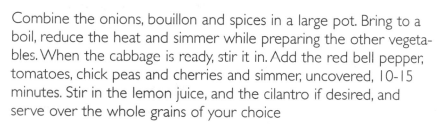

PEACHY CASSEROLE

4 cups bouillon
1 onion, chopped
4 cloves garlic, minced
1 green pepper, chopped
1 tablespoon oregano
pinch cayenne, to taste
1/4 cup white wine vinegar
1 28-ounce can tomatoes, undrained, broken up
1 pound winter squash,
1 pound red potatoes, cut in 1/2" chunks
1 pound sweet potatoes, cut in 1/2" chunks
2 cups corn
2 cups frozen peaches, cut in bite-size pieces
cooked whole grains

Pierce the squash with a knife in 2 or 3 places. Set in a microwave dish and microwave on high for 3 minutes or until it can be cut easily. When cool enough to handle, cut the squash in half and scoop out the seeds. Cut the squash into bite-size pieces; peel or not, as you wish.

Combine the bouillon, onion, garlic, pepper, oregano and cayenne in a large pot. Bring to a boil, reduce the heat and simmer while preparing the vegetables. Add the vinegar, tomatoes, squash, potatoes and sweet potatoes. Return to boiling, then reduce the heat and simmer, covered, about 20 minutes or until the potatoes are tender. Stir in the corn and peaches, adjust the seasoning and heat through. Serve over whole grains.

6-8 servings

CHUCKWAGON BEANS

1 onion, chopped
1 clove garlic, minced
1 cup canned tomato sauce
1 teaspoon bouillon granules or 1 bouillon cube
2 tart apples, cored and cut into bite-size pieces
1/4 cup dried cherries or golden raisins
1 teaspoon cinnamon
1/4 cup brown sugar, or to taste
2 tablespoons Worcestershire sauce
1/2 teaspoon liquid smoke flavoring, or to taste
3 cans (16 oz.) pink beans, undrained
Cooked kamut or other whole grains (optional)

Combine all ingredients except beans and whole grains in a large pot. Bring to a boil, reduce the heat and simmer, covered, 10 minutes (add a little bouillon if it gets too dry). Add the beans and simmer 10-15 minutes more. Serve over the whole grain of your choice.

6-8 servings

SOUTHWESTERN HOT POT

2 pounds winter squash
1 large onion, chopped
1/2 pound mushrooms, quartered or cut in 1/2" pieces
4 garlic cloves, minced
1 tablespoon mild chili powder
1 teaspoon thyme
1 teaspoon oregano
pinch cayenne, to taste
2 cups bouillon
1 red bell pepper, cut in 1/2" pieces
1 can pink beans or kidney beans, drained
2 cups frozen baby lima beans
2 cups frozen corn
2 tablespoons cider vinegar, or to taste
freshly ground black pepper
Cooked barley, kamut, or other whole grains of your choice

Pierce the squash with a knife in 2 or 3 places. Set in a microwave dish and microwave on high for 3 minutes. When cool enough to handle, cut the squash in half and scoop out the seeds. Return to the microwave and cook about 8 minutes more, or until you can easily scoop out the flesh.

Meanwhile, bring the onion, mushrooms, garlic, spices and bouillon to a boil in a large pot. Reduce the heat and simmer 5-10 minutes or until the onion is softened. Add the squash flesh, in bite-size pieces, along with the red pepper, pink beans and lima beans. Return to boiling, reduce the heat and simmer 5-10 minutes more, or until the lima beans are cooked. Stir in the corn and vinegar and adjust the seasonings. Serve over cooked whole grains.

6-8 servings

CURRIED LENTILS AND MUSHROOMS

1 cup lentils
1 onion, chopped
1 carrot, chopped
6 cups bouillon
1 tablespoon chopped fresh gingerroot
1 tablespoon mild curry powder
pinch cayenne, or to taste
1 pound fresh mushrooms
2 tablespoons lemon juice or vinegar

Bring the lentils, onion, carrot, bouillon and seasonings to a boil and simmer, uncovered, 30 minutes or until the lentils are tender and most of the liquid is absorbed. Cut the mushrooms in small pieces (removing the stems if they are tough.) Stir the mushrooms and lemon juice or vinegar into the lentils and cook, covered, 5-10 minutes.

4-6 servings

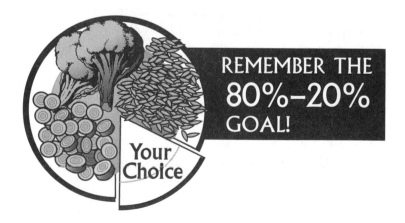

CIOPPINO

2 large onions, chopped
4 cloves garlic, minced
2 green peppers, or 1 green and 1 red, cut in 1/2" chunks
2-3 jalapeno peppers, seeded and chopped, to taste
3 stalks celery, chopped
2 cups bouillon or dry red wine, or some of each
1 28-ounce can Italian plum tomatoes, undrained, broken up
1 6-ounce can tomato paste
1 tablespoon oregano
3 small zucchini, halved lengthwise, then cut in 1/4" slices
3 pounds (total) seafood — your choice: shrimp, cleaned squid or
    any fish cut in 1" chunks, clams, mussels, scallops, etc.
1/2 cup chopped flat parsley
freshly ground black pepper, to taste
cooked whole grains of your choice (optional)

Combine the onions, garlic, peppers, celery and bouillon or wine in
a large pot. Bring to a boil, reduce the heat and simmer, covered, 10-
15 minutes. Stir in the tomatoes, tomato paste and spice blend and
cook 10 minutes more. Add the zucchini. Return the liquid to a boil
and add the seafood. Cover the pot, reduce the heat and cook, stirring once or twice, until the seafood is opaque (5-10 minutes.) Add
the parsley and black pepper; serve over whole grains if desired.

8-10 servings

PUCHERO (SMOKY STEW)

2 onions, chopped

2 cloves garlic, minced

3 mild fresh chiles, seeded and chopped (or use 2 green peppers and cayenne to taste)

2 cups bouillon

2 teaspoons ground cumin

2 tablespoons mild paprika

1/4 teaspoon liquid smoke

2 tablespoons tomato paste

4 medium potatoes, cut in chunks

2 carrots, sliced

1/2 pound portobello mushrooms, cut in chunks

1 16-ounce can pink beans or kidney beans, drained

1 bag frozen corn-black bean mixture or 2 cups frozen corn

1 package veggie pepperoni (optional)

Cooked barley or other whole grains of your choice

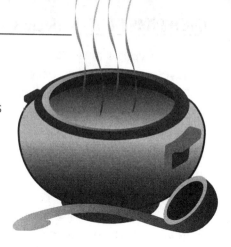

Combine the onions, garlic, chiles, bouillon and spices in a large pot. Bring to a boil, reduce the heat and simmer 10-15 minutes. Add the liquid smoke, tomato sauce, potatoes, carrots and mushrooms and simmer, covered, 20 minutes or more, until the vegetables are tender. Stir in the canned beans and the frozen corn-black bean mixture. If using the veggie pepperoni, cut it into bite-size pieces and drop into the stew. Heat through and serve over cooked whole grains.

6-8 servings

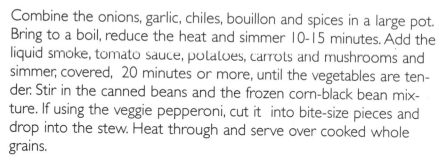

EASY VEGGIE BURGER CHILI

4 frozen veggie burgers
1 16-ounce bag frozen pepper-onion mix
1 28-ounce can crushed tomatoes
1 16-ounce can pink beans
1 16-ounce can chick peas
2 cups frozen corn
1 tablespoon mild chili powder
1 teaspoon ground cumin
pinch cayenne, to taste
Cooked barley or other whole grains of your choice

Break the veggie burgers into 1" chunks. Combine them with all of
the other ingredients in a large pot. Bring to a boil and simmer 5
minutes or more, until ready to serve. Ladle over the cooked whole
grains of your choice.

6-8 servings

SAUCY MUSHROOMS

1 cup dried mushrooms, broken in pieces, stems removed
2 cups boiling water
1 large onion, chopped
2 bouillon cubes or 2 teaspoons bouillon granules
1/2 cup water
1 pound fresh mushrooms, cut in bite-size pieces
1 red bell pepper, cut in 1/2" pieces
1 cup dry red wine
2 tablespoons Dijon-style mustard
2 tablespoons Worcestershire sauce
2 tablespoons brown sugar
1 tablespoon soy sauce
1 teaspoon or more freshly ground black pepper
1 12-ounce package tofu, cut in small cubes
Cooked wild rice or other whole grains of your choice
Chopped flat parsley or cilantro for garnish

Soak the dried mushrooms in the boiling water until softened, about 10 minutes.

Place the onion, bouillon paste and the 1/2 cup of water in a large pot and bring to a boil. Reduce the heat and cook until the onion is softened, about 5 minutes. Stir in the dried mushrooms and their soaking liquid, fresh mushrooms, red bell pepper, wine and seasonings. Return to boiling, mixing well. Reduce the heat and stir in the tofu. Simmer gently, uncovered, 30-40 minutes. Serve over whole grains, garnished with chopped parsley or cilantro.

4-6 servings

GIVETCH (ROUMANIAN VEGETABLE CASSEROLE)

2 onions, halved lengthwise, then sliced
1 clove garlic, minced
1 red bell pepper, cut in bite-size strips
1 green pepper, cut in bite-size strips
1 eggplant, cut in cubes
1 pound green beans, cut or broken in 2" pieces
2 carrots, sliced
4 medium red potatoes, cut in cubes
2 cups bouillon
1/4 cup tomato paste
2 tablespoons sweet paprika
generous pincy cayenne, to taste
1 teaspoon thyme
Salt and freshly ground black pepper to taste
Cooked whole grains of your choice

CHOOSE YOUR COOKING METHOD:
ON THE STOVETOP: put everything but the whole grains in a large pot, bring to a boil, reduce the heat to low, cover and simmer 30-45 minutes.

OVEN: Preheat to 375°, place everything but the whole grains in a covered casserole and bake about 1 hour.

SLOW COOKER: follow your unit's directions; cook 6-8 hours on low.

Cook until all of the vegetables are tender. Stir occasionally if you wish. Adjust the seasonings and serve over cooked whole grains (I add salt and black pepper at the table.)

You can add or subtract vegetables any way you wish. Add a can of kidney beans or chick peas for a heartier casserole. Good cold, too.

6-8 servings

ISLAND WILD RICE MEDLEY

1 onion, chopped
2 stalks celery, chopped
1 jalapeno pepper, seeded and minced
1/2 teaspoon cumin
1/2 teaspoon ground coriander
1/2 cup bouillon
2 cups cooked wild rice
2 cups cooked barley
1 red bell pepper, chopped
1 green pepper, chopped
1 16-ounce can black beans, rinsed and drained
1 ripe, fresh pineapple, peeled, cored and cut in 1/2" chunks (about 3 cups)
1/4 cup chopped cilantro

Cook the onion, celery, jalapeno pepper and spices in the bouillon until softened, 5-10 minutes. Stir in the remaining ingredients and heat through. Serve warm or at room temperature.

6-8 servings

PENANG SHRIMP CURRY

8 cups water
2 pounds shrimp
2 onions, chopped
1 clove garlic, minced
2 stalks celery, chopped
1 carrot, chopped
1 tart apple, cored and chopped
1 green pepper, chopped
4 bouillon cubes or 4 teaspoons bouillon granules
1/2 cup oatmeal
1 tablespoon curry powder
1/2 teaspoon nutmeg
pinch of cayenne, or to taste
1/2 cup chopped basil, mint or flat parsley, or some of each
Grated rind and juice of 1 lime
2 cups soy milk or light coconut milk
Cooked whole grains of your choice

Bring the water to a boil; add one pound of the shrimp and cook until it turns pink, about 3 minutes. Remove with a slotted spoon, return the liquid to boiling and cook the second pound the same way. Set the shrimp aside to cool. Let the water continue to boil until it is reduced to about 4 cups while you chop the vegetables.

Add the onion, garlic, celery, carrot, apple, green pepper, bouillon granules, oatmeal and seasonings to the water. Reduce the heat and simmer, uncovered, at least 30 minutes (more won't hurt).

Peel the shrimp. When ready to serve, stir in the shrimp, lime juice and soy or coconut milk and heat through. Ladle over cooked whole grains.

6-8 servings

EASY POTATO CURRY

6 medium red potatoes, cut in chunks
2 cups bouillon
1 16-ounce bag frozen pepper-onion mix
1 16-ounce bag frozen corn-black bean mix
1/2 pound portobello mushrooms, cut in chunks
2 cloves garlic or 2 teaspoons garlic paste
1 tablespoon mild curry powder
pinch cayenne, to taste
Cooked barley or other whole grains of your choice

Bring the potatoes and bouillon to a boil in a large pot. Reduce the heat and simmer 15-20 minutes, or until the potatoes are just tender. Add the frozen vegetables, mushrooms and seasonings; return to boiling, then reduce the heat and simmer 5-10 minutes. Add more bouillon if the mixture seems too dry. Serve over cooked whole grains.

4-6 servings

MEDITERRANEAN BEAN POT

1 large onion, chopped
1 red bell pepper, chopped
1 cup bouillon
1 cup white wine
2 cups canned tomato sauce or crushed tomatoes
1 teaspoon oregano
1 clove garlic, minced, or 1 teaspoon garlic paste
pinch cayenne or Tabasco sauce to taste
1 16-ounce can pink beans or white beans, drained
1 6-ounce can chopped clams, undrained
1/2 cup chopped fresh basil
Cooked barley or other whole grains of your choice

In a large pot, cook the onion and the pepper in the bouillon until soft, about 10 minutes. Add the remaining ingredients except the basil. Bring to a boil, reduce the heat and simmer 5-10 minutes to let the flavors blend. Stir in the basil and serve over whole grains.

6-8 servings

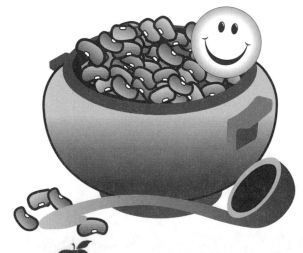

SPLIT PEA AND BARLEY STEW

1/2 cup uncooked barley
1 cup split peas
1 onion, chopped
2 cloves garlic, minced
4 cups bouillon
1 teaspoons cinnamon
1 teaspoon ground coriander
generous pinch cayenne, to taste
2 carrots, chopped
2 medium red potatoes, cut in 1/2" pieces
1/4 cup golden raisins
juice of 1 lemon
1/2 cup chopped Italian parsley
freshly ground black pepper
yogurt for garnish (optional)

Bring the barley, split peas, onion, garlic, bouillon and spices to a boil in a large pot. Reduce the heat, cover and simmer 30 minutes, stirring occasionally. Add the potatoes, carrots and raisins, return to boiling, reduce the heat and simmer about 30 minutes more, until the barley, split peas and vegetables are soft. Stir in the lemon juice and parsley, adjust the seasonings and add freshly ground black pepper to taste. Top each serving with a spoonful of yogurt if desired.

4-6 servings

LENTIL-VEGGIE LOAF

1 cup lentils
6 cups bouillon
1 cup chopped onion
1 cup chopped or shredded carrot
2 cups chopped mushrooms
1/2 cup bouillon
2 tablespoons tomato paste
1 tablespoon soy sauce
1 teaspoon sage
1 teaspoon oregano
pinch cayenne, to taste
1 cup quick-cooking oatmeal

Put the lentils and the 6 cups of bouillon in a pot; bring to a boil, reduce the heat and simmer 20-30 minutes, or until the lentils are tender. Drain, reserving about 1 cup of the cooking liquid.

Meanwhile, in another pot, cook the onion, carrot and mushrooms in 1/2 cup of bouillon until softened, about 5 minutes. Stir in the tomato paste, soy sauce, sage, oregano and cayenne.

Combine the lentils and the vegetable mixture. Stir in the oatmeal. You should have a stiff mixture; add a little of the reserved bouillon if necessary.

Spoon into a 9 x 5" microwaveable loaf pan and microwave on high for 10 minutes (or bake at 400° for 20 minutes.) Let cool for 5-10 minutes, then slice and serve.

6-8 servings

VARIATION: Shape the mixture into patties and grill on a hot non-stick pan.

BARBEQUE BEANS AND BARLEY

1 onion, chopped
2 cloves garlic, minced
1 can beer
1/2 cup ketchup
1/2 cup brown sugar
2 tablespoons Worcestershire sauce
1/2 teaspoon liquid smoke flavoring, or to taste
1/2 teaspoon cinnamon
2 cans pink beans, drained
2 cups cooked barley or other whole grain of your choice

Bring the onion, garlic, beer, ketchup, brown sugar and seasonings to a boil and boil gently 10 minutes or until thickened. Stir in the beans and barley, return to boiling and simmer 10 minutes more.

4-6 servings

FASTEST BEANS AND RICE

1 15-ounce can black beans
2 teaspoons bouillon granules
2 cups cooked brown rice or other whole grains
1 teaspoon mild chili powder
pinch cayenne, to taste
1/4 cup chopped Italian parsley or cilantro

Combine all ingredients, bring to a boil and simmer 3-5 minutes; or microwave for 3 minutes.

4-6 servings

QUICK VEGETABLE CURRY

2 16-ounce bags frozen mixed stir-fry vegetables
1/2 cup bouillon
1 tablespoon mild curry powder
pinch cayenne, or to taste
1 can chick peas
juice of one lime
2 cups light coconut milk or yogurt
Cooked whole grains of your choice
Bottled mango chutney (optional)

Combine the frozen vegetables, bouillon and spices in a large pot. Bring to a boil and simmer, covered, until they are crisp tender, 5-10 minutes (check your packages for suggested times.) Stir in the chick peas or beans and the lime juice. Add the coconut milk or yogurt; if using the yogurt, stir it in just before you serve the curry. Do not allow the mixture to boil after you add the yogurt. Serve over whole grains, with chutney on the side.

4 servings

VARIATION: Add shrimp or other seafood of your choice.

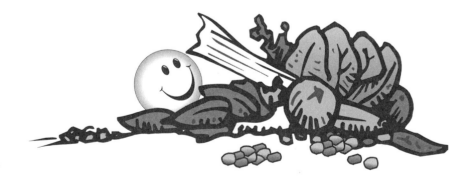

CREOLE BEANS 'N' GREENS

2 cups bouillon
1 16-ounce bag frozen onion-pepper mix
1 16-ounce bag frozen chopped kale or spinach
1 teaspoon liquid smoke
1 teaspoon Cajun Spice Blend
pinch cayenne, or to taste
2 tablespoons tomato paste
1 cup bulgur
1 can pinto or kidney beans
1/4 cup cider vinegar

Bring the bouillon, frozen vegetables and spices to a boil in a large pot, breaking up the vegetables with a spoon. Stir in the tomato paste and bulgur, return to boiling and simmer 5-10 minutes, or until the bulgur is soft. Stir in the beans and 2 tablespoons of the vinegar and heat through. Taste and add as much of the remaining vinegar as you like.

4 servings

EXTRA QUICK CHILI FOR DON IMUS

1 16-ounce bag frozen onion-pepper mix
2 garlic cloves, minced
1 28-ounce can plum tomatoes, cut in pieces
1 teaspoon bouillon granules
1 tablespoon mild chili powder
pinch cayenne, or to taste
2 cans kidney beans or black beans
Cooked whole grains (optional)

Combine all ingredients except the grains in a large pot, bring to a boil and simmer for 5-10 minutes. Serve over the whole grain of your choice, if desired.

4-6 servings

DR. GABE'S FAMOUS BEAN-EGGPLANT-TOMATO CASSEROLE

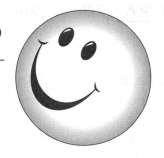

1 onion, chopped

2 cloves garlic, minced

1 green pepper, chopped

1 28-ounce can plum tomatoes, undrained, broken up

2 bouillon cubes or 2 teaspoons bouillon granules

1 tablespoon oregano

pinch cayenne, or to taste

1 eggplant, cut in 1/2" cubes

2 16-ounce cans kidney beans, drained

Cooked whole grains of your choice

Combine the onions, garlic, pepper, tomatoes, bouillon cubes or granules and seasonings in a large pot. Bring to a boil, reduce the heat and simmer while dicing the eggplant. Add eggplant to the pot and simmer 10-20 minutes. Stir in the beans and heat through. Serve over cooked whole grains.

6-8 servings

SOUPS

RED PEPPER SOUP

6 cups bouillon
1 onion, chopped
4 cloves garlic, minced
2 stalks celery, chopped
4 red bell peppers, cut in chunks
1 pound red potatoes, cut in chunks
1 tablespoon chili powder
pinch cayenne or Tabasco sauce, to taste

Combine all ingredients in a large pot. Bring to a boil, reduce the
heat and simmer 30-40 minutes, or until the vegetables are very
soft. Blend with a hand blender until smooth. Adjust the seasonings
and serve.

6-8 servings

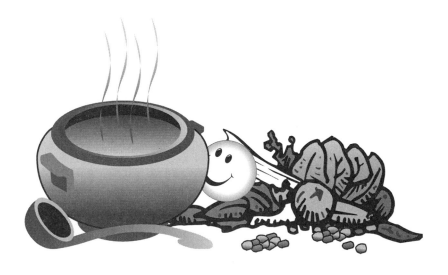

SPICY CHICKPEA SOUP

6 cups chicken bouillon
1 onion, chopped
4 cloves garlic, minced
1 carrot, chopped
2 stalks celery, chopped
2 red potatoes, cut in 1/2" cubes
1 teaspoon oregano
1-3 jalapeno peppers, seeded and minced, to taste
1 cup canned tomatoes, undrained, broken up
1 16-ounce can chickpeas, undrained
1 cup cooked kamut or other whole grain of your choice
1/4 cup chopped Italian parsley or cilantro
Freshly ground black pepper to taste

Combine all ingredients except the chickpeas, kamut and parsley in a large pot. Bring to a boil, reduce the heat and simmer, uncovered, 30-40 minutes or until the potatoes and carrot are tender. Whirl a hand blender in the soup for a few seconds to thicken it slightly, but leave lots of chunks. Stir in the chickpeas, kamut and parsley and cook about 10 minutes.

6-8 servings

LEMONY QUINOA SOUP

8 cups bouillon
1 onion, chopped
2 stalks celery, chopped
1 teaspoon oregano
1 teaspoon ground cumin
pinch cayenne, or to taste
1 cup quinoa
grated rind and juice of 2 lemons
1 16-ounce can artichoke hearts, drained
Lemon slices or wedges for garnish (optional)
Chopped fresh mint leaves (optional)

Bring the bouillon, onion and celery to a boil and simmer 10 minutes. Add the spices, quinoa and lemon rind and simmer 20-30 minutes, or until the quinoa is tender. Cut the artichoke hearts into bite-size pieces and add to the soup along with the lemon juice; simmer 5 minutes more. Serve garnished with lemon slices and mint leaves, if desired.

6-8 servings

YELLOW SPLIT PEA SOUP

8 cups bouillon
1 onion, chopped
2 cloves garlic, minced
2 teaspoons curry powder
1 teaspoon cinnamon
pinch cayenne, to taste
1 pound yellow split peas

Bring 1/2 cup of the bouillon to a boil in a large pot, stir in the onion, garlic and spices and cook together for 5 minutes. Add the remaining ingredients, bring to a boil and cook about 1 1/2 hours, or until the peas are very soft. Puree with a hand blender if you wish to make it very smooth.

6-8 servings

CHUNKY BLACK BEAN SOUP

2 onions, chopped
4 garlic cloves, minced
4 carrots, chopped
2 stalks celery, chopped
1 green pepper, chopped
1 jalapeno chile, seeded and minced, or to taste
2 teaspoons cumin
2 cups bouillon
2 16-ounce cans black beans, undrained
1 16-ounce can tomatoes, undrained, broken up
chopped cilantro for garnish (optional)

Combine the onions, garlic, carrots, celery, green pepper, jalapeno, cumin and bouillon in a large pot. Bring to a boil, reduce the heat and simmer, uncovered, 15-20 minutes or until the vegetables are soft. Add the beans and tomatoes and simmer 15-20 minutes more. Add more bouillon if you want a thinner soup.

6-8 servings

SALMON AND CORN BISQUE

1 onion, chopped
4 cups bouillon
2 medium red potatoes, cut into 1/2" chunks
1 teaspoon oregano
1/4 teaspoon thyme
pinch cayenne, or to taste
1/2 cup oatmeal
1/2 cup chopped red bell pepper
1 pound salmon steak or fillet, skinned and cut in 1-2" chunks
2 cups frozen or fresh corn
freshly ground black pepper to taste
paprika for garnish (optional)

Combine the onion, bouillion, potatoes, spices and oatmeal in a large pot. Bring to a boil, reduce the heat and simmer, uncovered, 15-20 minutes or until the potatoes are just tender. Puree briefly with the hand blender, but do not eliminate all chunks of potato. Add the red bell pepper and raise the heat just enough to return the soup to boiling. Stir in the salmon and corn, reduce the heat and simmer about 5 minutes, or until the largest salmon chunks are opaque in the center. Ladle into bowls and sprinkle with black pepper to taste and a pinch of paprika.

4-6 servings

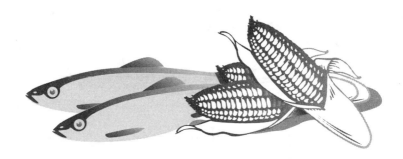

CREAMY CARROT SOUP

1 large onion, chopped
2 pounds carrots, chopped or shredded in a food processor
6 cups bouillon
1 tablespoon ground coriander
pinch cayenne, to taste
1 cup oatmeal
freshly ground black pepper to taste
chopped cilantro or Italian parsley
for garnish (optional)

Combine all ingredients, except the cilantro or parsley, in a large pot. Bring to a boil, reduce the heat and simmer, uncovered, 30-40 minutes. Use a hand blender to puree the soup until very smooth. Sprinkle each serving with cilantro or Italian parsley and more black pepper to taste.

4-6 servings

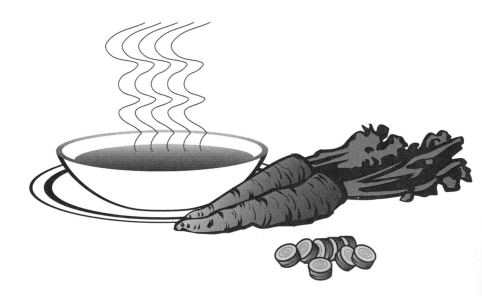

MUSHROOM BARLEY SOUP

8 cups bouillon
12 dried mushrooms, stems removed, broken in pieces
1 onion, chopped
2 cloves garlic, minced
1 teaspoon oregano
1/2 teaspoon thyme
pinch cayenne, or to taste
1/2 cup barley
2 medium red potatoes, cut in 1/2" cubes
1 8-ounce box mushrooms, quartered
1/2 cup chopped Italian parsley
2 tablespoons lemon juice, or to taste

Bring the bouillon to a boil in a large pot. Place the mushrooms in a small bowl and cover with 1 cup of the boiling bouillon; set aside to soak.

Add the onion, garlic, oregano, thyme, cayenne and barley potatoes to the pot and return to boiling. Reduce the heat and simmer for 30 minutes. Add the dried mushrooms and their soaking liquid, and the potatoes, and continue simmering until the barley and potatoes are tender. Add the fresh mushrooms and cook 10 minutes more. If you like a thick soup, puree briefly with the hand blender but leave lots of chunks. Stir in the parsley and lemon juice, adjust the seasonings and ladle into bowls.

6-8 servings

VIETNAMESE FISHERMAN'S SOUP

8 cups fish stock or bouillon
1 6" piece lemongrass, halved lengthwise and crushed
juice of one lime
4 cloves garlic, crushed in a garlic press
2 tablespoons Asian fish sauce (optional)
1 onion, halved and sliced thin
1 small hot green chile, seeded and sliced thin (optional)
1/2 pound catfish or any firm white fish, cut in 1" chunks
1/4 pound shrimp, steamed, peeled and sliced in half lengthwise
1 cup shredded Chinese cabbage
1 cup canned pineapple chunks and their juice
1 cup bean sprouts
1/4 cup chopped cilantro
8 cherry tomatoes, quartered

Bring the fish stock, lemon grass, lime juice, garlic, fish sauce, onion and chile to a boil and simmer 10 minutes. Remove the lemon grass. Add the fish; cook 3-4 minutes or until it is opaque. Add the shrimp and cook 2 minutes, or until they are pink. Stir in the remaining ingredients, cook 2 minutes more and serve immediately.

6-8 servings

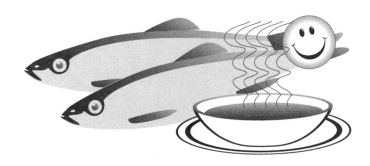

FALL VEGETABLE SOUP

6 cups bouillon
1 onion, chopped
4 cloves garlic, minced
2 stalks celery, chopped
2 carrots, cut in 1/4" slices
2 medium sweet potatoes, cut in 1/2" cubes
1 pound Brussels sprouts, halved or quartered
2 tablespoons tomato paste
2 tablespoons sweet paprika
1 teaspoon oregano
pinch cayenne, or to taste
1 16-ounce can black-eyed peas

Combine all ingredients except the black-eyed peas in a large pot. Bring to a boil, reduce the heat and simmer, covered, for 20-30 minutes, or until the sweet potatoes are very tender. Stir in the black-eyed peas, adjust the seasonings and serve in large bowls.

6-8 servings

GOLDEN SOUP

1 onion, chopped
3 cloves garlic, minced
1 tablespoon minced fresh gingerroot
4 cups bouillon
2 cups apple cider
1 tablespoon curry powder
1 teaspoon ground cumin
pinch of cayenne, to taste
1 cup orange lentils
4 carrots, sliced
4 parsnips, sliced
1 medium sweet potato, diced
juice of one lemon

OPTIONAL GARNISHES:
yogurt
chopped cilantro
chopped green onions

Bring the onion, garlic, gingerroot and ´ cup of the bouillon to a boil in a large pot. Reduce the heat and cook 5 minutes. Add the remaining ingredients except the lemon juice and return to boiling. Reduce the heat and simmer, uncovered, 20-30 minutes, or until the vegetables are soft and the lentils are tender but not mushy. Use a hand blender to thicken the soup a little, but do not puree smooth (you want some chunks and lentil bits.) Add the lemon juice, and serve with the garnishes of your choice.

6-8 servings

CREAMY CLAM CHOWDER

1 large onion, chopped
6 cups bouillon
1 medium cauliflower, chopped into florets
1 cup oatmeal (quick or rolled)
1 teaspoon oregano
pinch cayenne, or to taste
1 6.5-ounce can chopped clams, undrained
Freshly ground black pepper to taste

Combine the onion, bouillon, cauliflower, oats and spices in a pot and bring to a boil. Reduce the heat and simmer gently for 60 minutes, uncovered, stirring frequently. Allow to cool slightly. Puree the soup with a hand blender until smooth. Stir in the clams and their juice, adjust the seasonings to your taste and reheat. Serve with freshly ground black pepper.

4-6 servings

THREE SISTERS SOUP

The "Three Sisters" are corn, beans and squash, which were grown together by American Indians. The beans climbed on the corn stalks and returned nitrogen to the soil, and the low-growing squash vines shaded all the roots and kept weeds from sprouting. They can all be combined in one pot of delicious soup — with a recipe that uses three of everything!

3 pounds winter squash (such as acorn or hubbard)
3 onions, chopped
3 cups bouillon
3 teaspoons mild chili powder
3 small pinches cayenne, to taste
3 16-ounce cans white beans, undrained
3 cups fresh or frozen lima beans
3 cups frozen corn kernels
3 tablespoons chopped chives or green onions (optional)

Pierce the squash with a knife in 2 or 3 places. Set in a microwave dish and microwave on high for 3 minutes. When cool enough to handle, cut the squash in half and scoop out the seeds. Return to the microwave and cook about 5 minutes more, or until tender. Cut the squash into bite-size chunks, removing the skin.

Meanwhile, bring 1/2 cup of the bouillon to a boil, add the onions and cook 5-10 minutes. Stir in the rest of the bouillon, the chili powder and the white beans. Simmer gently until the squash is ready. Stir the squash into the soup. Mash the beans and squash slightly to thicken the soup, or use a hand blender. Add the lima beans and simmer 10 minutes or until the beans are tender. Stir in the corn, ladle the soup into bowls and garnish each serving with chopped chives or green onions, if desired.

6-8 servings

MEDITERRANEAN LIMA BEAN SOUP

2 onions, chopped
6 medium red potatoes, chopped
6 cups bouillon
1 teaspoon dried thyme
pinch cayenne, to taste
4 cups frozen baby lima beans
1 cup chopped cilantro or flat parsley
2 cups soy milk or yogurt
Roasted red peppers, cut in strips (optional)
Olives (preferably Greek-style), pitted and cut in chunks (optional)

Bring the onions, potatoes, bouillon, thyme and cayenne to a boil in a large pot. Reduce the heat and simmer 20 minutes. Add the lima beans and cilantro, return to boiling, then simmer 10 minutes more or until the potatoes are very tender. Stir in the soy milk or yogurt and heat through. Serve with freshly ground black pepper, garnished with red pepper strips and/or olives if desired.

6-8 servings

GREEN MINESTRONE

1 onion, chopped
2 stalks celery, chopped
8 cups bouillon
2 teaspoons oregano
pinch cayenne, or to taste
1/2 cup barley
1 medium red potato, cut in 1/2" cubes
4 cups chopped Swiss chard or spinach
2 small zucchini, cut in 1/2" chunks
1 16-ounce can chick peas
2 cups frozen green peas
1/2 cup chopped fresh basil or Italian parsley, or both
freshly ground black pepper, to taste

Combine the onion, celery, bouillon, oregano, cayenne and barley in a large pot. Bring to a boil, reduce the heat and simmer 30 minutes. Add the potato and cook 20-30 minutes more, or until the potato and barley are tender. Add the Swiss chard or spinach and the zucchini, return to a boil, then reduce the heat and simmer about 5 minutes or until the zucchini is tender but not mushy. Add the chick peas and green peas. Ladle into serving bowls, garnish with the chopped basil or parsley, and pass the pepper mill.

6-8 servings

SWEET POTATO BISQUE

1 onion, chopped
2 stalks celery, chopped
3 pounds sweet potatoes, peeled if necessary and diced
8 cups bouillon
1 tablespoon mild curry powder
2 teaspoons thyme
1 teaspoon freshly ground black or white pepper
pinch cayenne, to taste
1/4 cup brandy (optional)
2 cups soy milk or light coconut milk

Combine the onion, celery, sweet potatoes, bouillon, curry powder and peppers in a large pot. Bring to a boil, reduce the heat and simmer, 30-40 minutes, or until the potatoes are soft. With a slotted spoon, remove about 2 cups of the vegetables and set aside. Puree the remaining soup with a hand blender until smooth. Return the vegetables to the pot, stir in the brandy and soy milk or cocunut milk, and heat through.

6-8 servings

MOROCCAN CHICK PEA SOUP

1/2 cup bulgur
6 cups bouillon
2 15-ounce cans chick peas
2 teaspoons oregano
1/4 teaspoon harissa, or to taste (see page 106)
1 bag spinach, chopped, or 1 box frozen chopped spinach, thawed
Lemon slices or wedges for garnish

Bring the bulgur and 5 cups of the bouillon to a boil. Meanwhile, place the remaining cup of bouillon and one can of the chick peas in blender; puree until smooth. Add them to the pot, along with the other can of chick peas, the spices and spinach. Return to boiling, them simmer until the bulgur is soft, 5-10 minutes. Serve with lemon wedges.

4-6 servings

MARYLAND CRAB SOUP

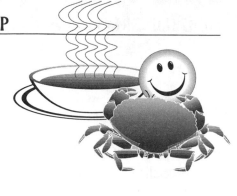

1 onions, chopped
2 cloves garlic, minced
1 green pepper, chopped
3 stalks celery, chopped
6 cups bouillon
1 29-ounce can tomato sauce
1 bay leaf
1 teaspoon oregano
pinch of cayenne (to taste)
2 potatoes, diced
2 carrots, sliced
1 cups fresh or frozen corn kernels
1/2 pound crab meat
1/2 cup Italian parsley, chopped
Freshly ground black pepper

Cook the onions, garlic, green pepper and celery in 1/2 cup of the bouillon to soften, 5-10 minutes. Add the remaining bouillon, tomato sauce, bay leaf, oregano, red peppers, potatoes and carrots and cook 20 minutes, or until the vegetables are tender. Stir in the corn, crabmeat and parsley and simmer 5 minutes. Serve with ground pepper to taste.

6-8 servings

DOUBLE GREEN PEA SOUP

1 cup split peas
6 cups bouillon
2 onions, chopped
4 cloves garlic, minced
2 teaspoons oregano or Italian Spice Blend
pinch cayenne pepper, or more to taste
1/2 cup bulgur
1 28-ounce can Italian plum tomatoes, undrained, broken up
1 pound spinach, torn in pieces, or one box frozen spinach, thawed
Freshly ground black pepper to taste

Bring the split peas and bouillon to a boil in a large pot and cook 20 minutes, or until they are just barely tender. Add the onions, garlic, seasonings, bulgur and tomatoes and simmer 20-30 minutes. Put the spinach on top of the mixture, cover the pot and simmer just until spinach wilts, about 2 minutes. Stir the spinach in and serve in bowls with ground pepper to taste.

6-8 servings

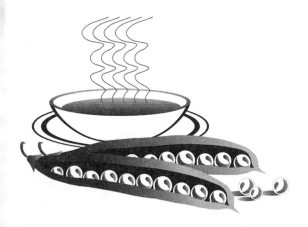

HOT AND SOUR MUSHROOM SOUP

6 cups bouillon
1 6" piece lemongrass, split lengthwise and crushed
Rind of one lemon, grated
2 garlic cloves, minced
1/2 cup bamboo shoots cut in matchsticks
1 bunch green onions, sliced thin
1/2 pound mushrooms, sliced
2 tablespoons oyster sauce
2 tablespoons cornstarch
2 tablespoons water
juice of one lemon
1/2 teaspoon chili paste, or a pinch of cayenne, to taste
1/4 cup chopped cilantro

In a large pot, bring the bouillon, lemon grass, lemon rind, garlic and; simmer, covered, 15-20 minutes. Add the bamboo shoots, green onions, mushrooms and oyster sauce and cook 5 minutes. Mix the cornstarch and water into a smooth paste and stir into the soup; return the soup to a boil. Remove the lemon grass, stir in the lemon juice and add chili paste or cayenne to taste. Ladle into soup bowls and garnish with the cilantro.

4-6 servings

FESTIVE SHRIMP CHOWDER

8 cups bouillon
1 pound shrimp
6 cloves garlic, minced
4 green onions, chopped
2 jalapeno chiles, seeded
and chopped, or to taste
1/2 teaspoon nutmeg
2 potatoes, cut in 1/2" dice
1 cup cooked barley or brown rice
3 cups frozen corn
2 cups frozen peas
2 cups soy milk or light coconut milk
Freshly ground black pepper to taste
Chopped cilantro or flat parsley for garnish (optional)
Lime wedges

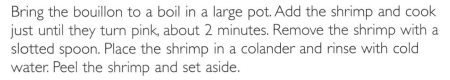

Bring the bouillon to a boil in a large pot. Add the shrimp and cook just until they turn pink, about 2 minutes. Remove the shrimp with a slotted spoon. Place the shrimp in a colander and rinse with cold water. Peel the shrimp and set aside.

Meanwhile, add the garlic, green onions, chiles, nutmeg and potatoes to the bouillon. Bring the soup back up to a boil, then reduce the heat and simmer until the potatoes are just tender, about 15 minutes. Stir in the barley and frozen corn and bring back to boiling again. Reduce the heat; stir in the frozen peas, soy milk and reserved shrimp. Heat through and adjust the seasonings. Garnish with cilantro or parsley if desired and serve with lime wedges.

6-8 servings

HARIRA

1 large onion, chopped
1 red bell pepper chopped
2 stalks celery, chopped
2 cloves garlic, chopped
8 cups bouillon
1 cup lentils
1 28-ounce can Italian plum tomatoes, undrained, broken up
1/2 teaspoon Harissa, (see page 106) or hot sauce, to taste
1 can chick peas
1/2 cup chopped Italian parsley
juice of 1 lemon (about 1/4 cup)
cooked whole grains (optional)
lemon wedges
freshly ground black pepper, to taste

In a large pot, cook the onion, green pepper, celery and garlic in 1/2 cup of bouillon until softened, 5-10 minutes. Stir in the lentils and the remaining bouillon and bring to a boil. Reduce the heat to a simmer, add the tomatoes and harissa and cook until the lentils are tender, 25-30 minutes. Add the chick peas, parsley and lemon juice. If you wish, stir in a cup or two of cooked whole grains or place 1/2 cup of grains in the bottom of each serving bowl. Serve with lemon wedges and freshly ground black pepper.

6-8 servings

SALADS

SPICY CRAB SALAD

1/2 pound crab meat
1 cup cherry tomatoes, halved or quartered
2 stalks celery, chopped fine (use tender inner stalks)
1/4 cup chopped fresh basil leaves
1/4 cup chopped cilantro leaves
1 teaspoon mild chile powder
1 jalapeno chile, seeded and minced
2 cups cooked, chilled barley
1/4 cup lime juice, to taste

Combine all ingredients and chill.

4-6 servings

QUINOA-CARROT SALAD

2 cups cooked, chilled quinoa
4 cups shredded carrots (use food processor)
2 cups finely chopped Italian parsley
1/4 cup lemon juice
1 clove garlic, minced
freshly ground black pepper to taste

Combine all ingredients and chill.

4-6 servings

GREEK OLIVE SALAD

1/4 cup lemon juice
1 clove garlic, minced
1/2 teaspoon oregano
2 cups cooked, chilled barley or other whole grain of your choice
1/2 cucumber, chopped
1 cup cherry tomatoes, halved or quartered
1 red bell pepper, chopped
2 green onions, chopped
1 14-ounce can artichokes, drained and cut in bite-size pieces
1/4 cup chopped Italian parsley
8-12 pitted black Greek olives, sliced or chopped
freshly ground black pepper to taste

Combine the lemon juice, garlic and oregano and stir into the grains. Add the remaining ingredients and chill.

4-6 servings

ASIAN ASPARAGUS SALAD

For the dressing:

1/4 cup rice vinegar
2 cloves garlic, minced in a garlic press
2 tablespoons soy sauce
1 tablespoon grated fresh gingerroot
1/2 teaspoon Tabasco or other hot sauce, or to taste

For the salad:

1 pound asparagus
1 red bell pepper, chopped
2 stalks celery, chopped
1 cup canned baby corns, drained
2 cups cooked barley, brown rice or
    other whole grains of your choice

Combine the dressing ingredients.

Break the tough ends off the asparagus and cut the stalks into 1"
pieces. (Diagonal cuts look attractive.) Steam the asparagus for 8
minutes, or until just crisp-tender. (Alternatively, cook in boiling
water for 3-4 minutes.) Rinse the cooked asparagus in cold water
and drain.

Combine the asparagus with the remaining salad ingredients and
stir in the dressing.

4-6 servings

BEAN SALAD WITH SMOKED SALMON

1/4 pound smoked salmon, cut in bite-size pieces
1 16-ounce can small white beans , drained
2 oranges, peeled and cut in bite-size pieces
1 small red onion, chopped
2 stalks celery, chopped
1 jalapeno chili, seeded and minced, or to taste
1 cup frozen green peas
1/2 cup Italian parsley, chopped
1 teaspoon oregano
juice of one lemon or 2 tablespoons red wine vinegar
2 tablespoons fat-free Italian dressing, or to taste

Mix all ingredients except the Italian dressing. Taste and decide
whether you want the additional moisture (some smoked salmon is
dry, some is moist) and add the dressing as desired. Chill.

4-6 servings

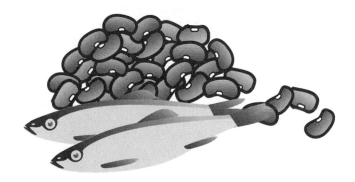

CITRUS-WALDORF SALAD

2 tart apples, cored and cut in chunks
2 oranges or 6 tangerines, peeled and cut in bite-size pieces
1 bell pepper, chopped
1 stalk celery, chopped
1 bunch green onions, sliced
1/2 cup golden raisins
1 8-ounce can sliced water chestnuts, drained
1 cup cooked, chilled wild rice
juice of 1 lemon
1/2 cup fat-free mayonnaise
1/2 teaspoon cinnamon or dessert spice blend

Combine all ingredients and chill.

4-6 servings

NEW POTATO SALAD

For the salad:

1 pound tiny red new potatoes
1 cup cooked, chilled quinoa or other whole grains
1 red bell pepper, chopped
2 stalks celery, chopped
1 bunch green onions, sliced
1/2 cup chopped Italian parsley

For the dressing:

1/2 cup fat-free mayonnaise, yogurt or a combination of the two
2 tablespoons Dijon mustard
2 tablespoons balsamic vinegar
2 teaspoons fennel seeds
Freshly ground black pepper, to taste

Cook the potatoes in boiling water to cover for 10-15 minutes or until just tender. Drain and rinse with cold water to stop the cooking. Cut into bite-size pieces. Combine the potatoes with the remaining salad ingredients and chill. Combine the dressing ingredients. When ready to serve, stir the dressing into the salad.

4-6 servings

ZESTY LENTIL SALAD

1/2 cup red lentils
1/2 cup small green (French) lentils
4 cups bouillon
1/4 cup balsamic vinegar
2 cloves garlic, minced
1-2 fresh hot chiles, seeded and minced, to taste
1 cup cooked, chilled wild rice or other whole grains
2 ripe tomatoes, cut in 1/2" chunks
1 bunch green onions
1/4 cup chopped cilantro or Italian parsley

Bring the lentils and the bouillon to a boil; reduce the heat and simmer until the lentils are just tender, about 20 minutes. Drain off any excess liquid and run cold water over them to stop the cooking. Drain.

Meanwhile, combine the vinegar, garlic and minced chile. When the lentils are ready, combine them with the vinegar mixture and the remaining ingredients. Chill until ready to serve.

4-6 servings

BARLEY-FRUIT SALAD
WITH CHUTNEY DRESSING

2 cups cooked barley
1 bunch green onions, sliced
1 teaspoon curry powder
2 tart apples, cored and diced
1 cup crushed pineapple, drained
1/4 cup dried apricots, chopped
1/4 cup chopped mint or cilantro, or some of each
1/4 cup mango chutney
1/2 cup plain or vanilla yogurt or 1/4 cup plain or vanilla soy milk

Combine all ingredients and chill.

4-6 servings

PINEAPPLE-BLACK BEAN SALAD

1/2 fresh pineapple, cut in 1/2" chunks (about 2 cups)
1 16-ounce can black beans, drained and rinsed
2 cups cooked, chilled barley
1/4 cup rice vinegar, or to taste
1/2 cup chopped cilantro
1 tablespoon hot red pepper relish, or to taste

Combine all ingredients and chill.

4-6 servings

LATIN QUINOA SALAD

2 cups cooked quinoa
1 cucumber, seeded and chopped
1 cup frozen corn
1 cup frozen peas
1 red bell pepper, chopped
1-2 jalapeno peppers, seeded and minced, to taste
1/4 cup chopped cilantro or Italian parsley
juice of 2 limes
Freshly ground black pepper, to taste

Combine all ingredients and chill.

4-6 servings

BLACK BEAN-WILD RICE SALAD

1 16-ounce can black beans, drained and rinsed
2 cups cooked wild rice
1 14-ounce can artichoke hearts, drained and quartered
1/2 cup roasted red peppers or pimentoes, cut in 1/2" pieces
1/2 cup chopped red onion
1/2 cup chopped cilantro or flat parsley
1 teaspoon chile powder
pinch cayenne, to taste
1/4 cup fat free Italian dressing, or enough to moisten

Combine all ingredients and chill.

4-6 servings

SWEET POTATO-CRANBERRY SALAD

2 pounds sweet potatoes, cut in 1/2" chunks
1 small red onion, chopped
1 stalk celery, chopped
1/2 cup dried cranberries
1 tablespoon Dijon-style mustard
2 tablespoons mango chutney
1/4 cup vanilla soy milk or yogurt
2 tablespoons cider vinegar

Steam the sweet potatoes until they are just tender, about 15-20 minutes. As soon as they are done, rinse them with cold water to stop the cooking and drain.

Meanwhile, combine the other ingredients in a serving bowl. When the sweet potatoes are ready, mix them in. Chill until ready to serve.

4-6 servings

FRUITY KAMUT SALAD

2 cups cooked, chilled kamut or wheat berries
2 apples, cored and cut in 1/2" chunks
2 oranges, cut in bite-size pieces
2 cups fresh pineapple, cut in 1/2" chunks
1 small fennel bulb, halved lengthwise, then sliced crosswise about 1/4" wide
1/4 cup chopped Italian parsley
1/4 cup fat-free mayonnaisde
1 tablespoon Dijon mustard
2 tablespoons lemon juice
1 teaspoon fennel seeds

Combine all ingredients. If you make this ahead, stir in the mayonnaise just before serving.

4-6 servings

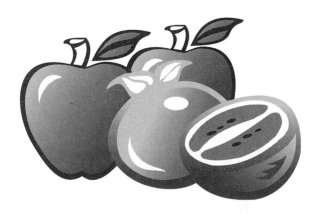

MIXED GRAINS SALAD
WITH ARTICHOKES

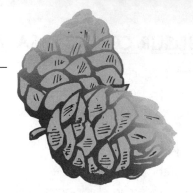

1 16-ounce can artichoke hearts
1/4 cup fat-free Italian
    salad dressing
1 clove garlic, minced
1 green pepper, chopped
1 bunch green onions, sliced thin
1/2 cup sliced stuffed green olives
2 cups cooked, chilled barley or other whole grain of your choice
1 cup cooked wild rice
1 1/2 teaspoons curry powder
1/2 cup fat-free mayonnaise

Drain the artichoke hearts and cut them into bite size pieces. Place them in a small dish with the salad dressing and the garlic and let marinate at least 30 minutes, stirring occasionally. Combine with the remaining ingredients. If you make this ahead, stir in the mayonnaise just before serving.

6-8 servings

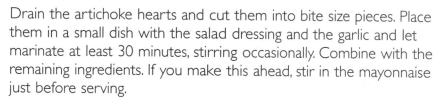

BULGUR CONFETTI SALAD

1 cup bulgur
1 1/2 cups boiling bouillon
3 broccoli stalks (save the florets for another use)
3 medium carrots
1 red onion, chopped fine
1 cup chopped flat parsley
1 16-ounce can chick peas, drained
2 tablespoons lemon juice
1/4 cup fat-free Italian dressing, or enough to moisten

Place the bulgur and the boiling bouillon in a bowl and let stand until the bulgur is soft, 20-30 minutes. Drain off any excess liquid.

Meanwhile, shred the broccoli stalks and the carrots in a food processor. Combine the shredded vegetables and the remaining ingredients with the softened bulgur and chill.

4-6 servings

FENNEL SALAD WITH CLEMENTINES

1 large or 3 small fennel bulbs
10 clementines or tangerines
1/4 cup lemon juice
2 tablespoons fennel seeds
1 teaspoon ground cumin
1 clove garlic, minced
pinch cayenne, or to taste
1/2 teaspoon salt, or to taste
Freshly ground black pepper to taste

Trim the fennel bulbs, discarding the base and stems. Cut the bulb in quarters lengthwise and then slice crosswise into 1/4" slices. If the feathery tops look fresh, chop them and add to the sliced pieces.

Peel the clementines, cut them in half crosswise and separate them into sections. Mix all but 1/2 cup of the clementine sections with the fennel in a serving bowl.

Make the dressing: Crush the remaining 1/2 cup of the clementine sections with the back of a spoon. Add the lemon juice and seasonings. Combine with the fennel and clementines and let sit for at least 1 hour to blend the flavors.

4-6 servings

HOLIDAY WILD RICE SALAD

4 cups cooked wild rice
1 cup dried cranberries
1/4 cup finely chopped red onion
1 6-ounce can water chestnuts, drained and chopped
1 cup crushed pineapple, drained
1/2 cup chopped basil or flat parsley
1/2 cup rice vinegar, or to taste

Combine all ingredients and chill. **4-6 servings**

LENTIL-MINT SALAD

1 cup lentils, preferably tiny green French lentils
6 cups bouillon
2 tablespoons lemon juice
1/2 teaspoon ground cumin
1/2 cup finely chopped red onion
1 red bell pepper, cut in 1/2" chunks
1/2 cup chopped mint

Combine the lentils and bouillon in a pot. Bring to a boil, reduce the heat and simmer for 20-30 minutes, or until the lentils are tender but still firm (do not let them get mushy.) Drain the lentils, reserving about 1/4 cup of the bouillon. Rinse the lentils with cold water to cool.

Combine the drained lentils with the remaining ingredients. Add a little of the reserved bouillon if the mixture seems too dry. Serve at room temperature or chilled.

4-6 servings

SEPTEMBER SALAD

2 cups cooked quinoa
1 cup frozen corn
1 16-ounce can pink beans, drained and rinsed
1 vine-ripened tomato, chopped
1 bunch green onions, chopped
1/4 cup chopped cilantro or Italian parsley
juice of 1 lemon
1 teaspoon mild chili powder or ground cumin
tabasco sauce to taste

Combine all ingredients. Serve with the bottle of hot sauce on the side, so each diner can add more heat to his or her taste.

4-6 servings

MANGO SALAD WITH BARLEY AND BEANS

1 small red onion, chopped
2 mangoes, peeled and chopped
1 can black beans, drained and rinsed
2 cups cooked, chilled barley
1/2 cup chopped cilantro or Italian parsley
1/4 cup rice vinegar, or 1/2 cup grapefruit juice, to taste
1 teaspoon ground cumin
1-2 jalapeno chiles, seeded and chopped, or to taste

Combine all ingredients and chill.

4-6 servings

CURRIED WILD RICE SALAD

2 cups cooked wild rice
1/2 cup golden raisins
1/2 cup green pepper, chopped
1 cup seedless grapes
1 bunch green onions, sliced
1/4 cup chopped Italian parsley
2 tablespoons lemon juice
1 teaspoon mild curry powder
1/2 cup no-fat mayonnaise, or enough to moisten grains

Combine all ingredients. If you make this ahead, stir in the mayonnaise just before serving.

4 servings

THAI SLAW

4 cups shredded Napa or Chinese cabbage
1 cup shredded carrots
1/2 red onion, sliced thin
1 cup pineapple tidbits, drained
1/4 cup rice wine vinegar
1 tablespoon Asian fish sauce (optional)
1/4 cup chopped cilantro

Combine all ingredients and chill.

4 servings

CHEROKEE SALAD

2 cups cooked wild rice
1 cup frozen corn
1 16-ounce can small red beans, drained and rinsed
1 red bell pepper, chopped
1 bunch green onions, chopped
1/4 cup chopped cilantro, chopped
1/4 cup rice vinegar or lemon juice, to taste
1 teaspoon mild chili powder
tabasco sauce to taste

Combine all ingredients.

4-6 servings

CAESAR TOFU DRESSING

2 garlic cloves, peeled and minced
1 tablespoon Dijon mustard
12-ounce package of tofu
2 tablespoons Asian fish sauce or soy sauce
1/4 cup lemon juice
1 teaspoon freshly ground black pepper

Combine all ingredients in a blender and puree until smooth. Keeps well.

YIELD: about 1 cup

Note: Toss into a bowl of romaine lettuce or your favorite salad greens. Add a little shredded romano or parmesan cheese and some anchovies (if you like) for a delicious Caesar salad.

DESSERTS, SNACKS & CONDIMENTS

ORANGE DESSERT GRAINS

6 oranges

2 cups cooked oat groats, barley or quinoa, warm or at room temperature

1/4 cup orange marmalade

2 tablespoons orange liqueur such as Grand Marnier or Sabra (optional)

1/4 teaspoon cinnamon

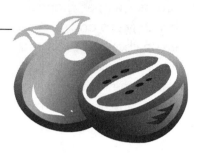

Grate the rind of one of the oranges into a mixing bowl. Peel the oranges, section them and cut the sections into small bite-size pieces, working so any juice runs into the mixing bowl. Add the remaining ingredients and mix well.

4-6 servings

FALL FRUIT CURRY

1 cup bouillon
1 teaspoon curry powder
1 teaspoon dessert spice blend or cinnamon
1 tablespoon grated fresh ginger
2 tablespoons brown sugar, or to taste
4 tart apples, cored and cut in bite-size pieces
2 pears, cored and cut in bite-size pieces
2 cups fresh or frozen peaches, cut in bite size pieces
1 cup fresh or canned pineapple, bite-size
1/2 cup dried cherries or cranberries
cooked barley or other whole grains (optional)

Combine the bouillon, curry powder, dessert blend, ginger and brown sugar in a large pot. Bring to a boil, reduce the heat and simmer about 5 minutes to blend the flavors. Add the fruits, cover and simmer until the fruits are soft and a little syrupy, about 20 minutes. Serve over whole grains or mix into grains if desired.

6-8 servings

CARROT KHEER (INDIAN RICE PUDDING)

4 cups shredded carrots (use a food processor)
1 cup bouillon
2 cups cooked oat groats or barley
1 cup soy milk
1/2 cup golden raisins
2 tablespoons brown sugar, or to taste
1/2 teaspoon dessert spice blend

Bring the carrots and bouillon to a boil in a medium saucepan and cook, stirring, about 10 minutes or until the carrots are soft. Drain off any excess bouillon. Stir in the remaining ingredients and cook over low heat for 5-10 minutes. Serve warm or chilled.

4-6 servings

GRAPEFRUIT COMPOTE WITH RUM CHERRIES

1/4 cup rum
1/4 cup water(or use 1/2 cup water and 1 teaspoon rum extract)
1/2 cup dried cherries
1/2 teaspoon cinnamon or dessert spice blend
3 large or 6 small grapefruit

Place the rum, water, cherries and cinnamon or spice blend in a small pan or microwave dish. Bring to a boil, remove from the heat, stir and let stand while preparing the grapefruit.

Peel and section the grapefruit and remove excess white pith, and the membranes if desired. Cut each segment into bite-size pieces. Place in a serving bowl and stir in the cherry mixture.

4-6 servings

NOT-A-FRUITCAKE

4 medium beets
2 medium sweet potatoes
1/2 cup dried cranberries
1/2 cup dried apricots, cut in small pieces
1/2 cup golden raisins
1/2 cup dried pineapple tidbits, cut in small pieces
1/4 cup candied ginger, diced into tiny pieces
1/2 cup rum, brandy or fruit juice
2 cups cooked quinoa or barley
1 cup quick-cooking oatmeal
1/2 cup brown sugar
1 teaspoon dessert spice blend or cinnamon
1 teaspoon vanilla extract
12 chestnuts, peeled and cut in small pieces
1/2 cup Egg Beaters or other liquid egg substitute

Preheat the oven to 375°

Trim the ends off the beets and sweet potatoes, cut them into 1/2" chunks and steam until very tender, about 30 minutes. Drain.

Meanwhile, combine the dried fruits and rum or other liquid of your choice in a small bowl and allow them to soak.

Place the cooked beets and sweet potatoes in a bowl and mash them together. Stir in the dried fruits and their soaking liquid and all the remaining ingredients and mix thoroughly. Spoon the mixture into a non-stick loaf pan. Bake at 375° for 1 1/2 hours. Allow to cool before slicing. Serve at room temperature or chilled.

8-10 servings

CREAMY APPLE DESSERT

2 large or 4 small apples, cored and cut in chunks
1/2 cup raisins
1/2 teaspoon dessert spice blend
2 tablespoons sugar (optional)
2 tablespoons rum or water
2 cups cooked barley or quinoa
1 cup vanilla-flavored soy milk
1/4 cup quick oatmeal

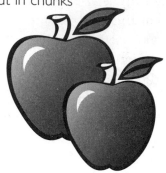

Combine the apples, raisins, spice, sugar and rum or water in a microwaveable bowl. Cover and microwave on high for 6-8 minutes, stirring once or twice, until the apples are soft. Add the remaining ingredients and microwave 3-4 minutes more.

4 servings

MICROWAVE PUMPKIN PUDDING

2 cups canned pumpkin puree (unsweetened)
1/2 cup brown sugar
2 teaspoons grated or minced fresh
  gingerroot
1/2 teaspoon cinnamon
juice and grated rind of 1 lemon
1/2 cup quick-cooking oatmeal
1/2 cup liquid egg substitute

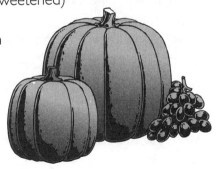

Combine the pumpkin, sugar, gingerroot, cinnamon, lemon juice and
lemon rind in a large microwave dish. Cook on high 4 minutes, stirring once or twice. Stir in the oatmeal and egg substitute and let
the mixture sit for 5 minutes. Cover loosely, return to the
microwave and cook 3 minutes, turning the dish once or twice.
Serve warm, at room temperature or chilled, dusted with a little
cinnamon if you wish.

4 servings

BANANA RICE PUDDING

2-4 ripe bananas, sliced
2 cups cooked brown rice, barley or oat groats
2 tablespoons brown sugar
1/4 teaspoon vanilla extract
1/4 teaspoon dessert spice blend or cinnamon

Combine all ingredients in a microwaveable dish and microwave on
high for 3-4 minutes, or until the bananas are soft and the grains
are heated through. Stir and serve.

4-6 servings

MANGO SORBET

1 large ripe (very sweet) mango, skin and seed removed
1 cup water
1 tablespoon minced candied ginger (optional)

Combine all ingredients in a blender and puree until smooth. Taste; if it is not sweet enough, add sugar or sweetener.

Pour into the bowl of an ice cream freezer and freeze according to your machine's instructions. Or pour into a small metal bowl and place in your freezer; stir every 20 minutes or so until the mixture is soft-frozen.

4 servings

BANANA-PINEAPPLE ICE

Note: whenever you have ripe (not black) bananas that you can't use up fast enough, peel them, wrap them in saran wrap or put in baggies, and put in your freezer. You can use them in fruit smoothies or this instant dessert!

4 frozen bananas
1 cup canned crushed pineapple with its juice

Whirl the bananas and pineapple in the blender and serve.

4 servings

BEAN-PEPPER SALSA

1 16-ounce can small red beans
1 10-ounce can shoepeg corn
2-4 tablespoons hot red pepper relish, or to taste
1 bunch green onions, white part only, sliced thin
1 red bell pepper, seeded and chopped

Mix all ingredients together and chill.

Yield: About 3 cups

BLACK-EYED PEA RELISH

1 16-ounce can black-eyed peas
1 large sweet Vidalia or red onion, chopped fine
1 red bell pepper, chopped
2 stalks celery, chopped
1 tablespoon hot red pepper relish, or to taste
1/4 cup cider vinegar
2 tablespoons prepared Dijon mustard
1/2 teaspoon whole mustard seed (optional)

Combine all ingredients and chill.

Yield: About 3 cups

MOROCCAN ORANGE-ONION CONDIMENT

6 oranges
1 large red onion, chopped
12 olives (green or black), pitted and sliced
1/4 teaspoon Harissa sauce (see page XX) or hot sauce, to taste

Peel the oranges and slice them crosswise. Mix the remaining ingredients and stir them into the orange slices. Let sit at least 20 minutes, or refrigerate until ready to serve.

Yield: About 4 cups

ZIPPY BLACK BEAN DIP

1 can black beans, drained
1 clove garlic
2 pickled jalapeno peppers (or more to taste)
1 tablespoon red wine vinegar
2 teaspoons Worcestershire sauce
1 teaspoon chili powder

Mash the ingredients together or puree in a blender. Serve with raw vegetable dippers.

Yield: About 2 cups

SPICY PEANUT DIP

You can make this as zippy or mild as you like, depending on the heat of your favorite salsa. Add Tabasco sauce to your taste if you want to turn up the heat.

1 cup crunchy style peanut butter
1 cup medium-hot salsa
2 tablespoons brown sugar
1/4 cup lemon juice
2 tablespoons worcestershire sauce

Combine all ingredients in a bowl, using a fork to mash up any chunks of salsa. Serve with raw veggies.

Yield: About 2 cups

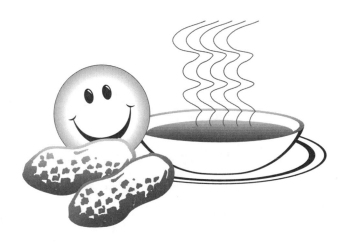

DOUBLE MUSHROOM GRAVY

8 dried mushrooms, stems removed,
broken in pieces

2 cups hot bouillon

1/2 pound fresh mushrooms,
chopped

3 tablespoons soy sauce

2 tablespoons cornstarch dissolved in
1/4 cup cold water

freshly ground black pepper

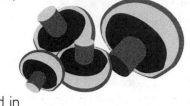

Cover the mushroom pieces with the hot bouillon in a blender container. Let soak 20 minutes. When the mushrooms are soft, run the blender briefly to chop them fine.

Pour the mushroom-bouillon mixture into a pot and bring to a boil. Add the fresh mushrooms and soy sauce; cook 5-10 minutes. Stir in the cornstarch-water mixture and continue to cook 2-3 minutes, until thickened. Season with black pepper to taste.

Yield: About 2 cups

WILD RICE WITH DRIED CHERRIES

Here's a simple, festive side dish that's a favorite in our house.

4 cups cooked wild rice
1/2 cup dried cherries

Mix the cherries into the wild rice while it's still hot, or heat them together in the microwave.

4 servings

MICROWAVE CHUTNEY

2 chopped fruit (your choice — tart apples, mangoes, peaches, pineapple, etc., or a combination)
1 onion, chopped
1 cup raisins, currants or chopped dates, or a combination
1/2 cup cider vinegar
1 tablespoon minced fresh ginger
1/2 teaspoon dessert spice blend or cinnamon
1 teaspoon mustard seeds
1 teaspoon fennel seeds
pinch cayenne, to taste

Combine all ingredients in a large microwaveable bowl. Microwave on high for 15 minutes, stirring every 3-5 minutes.

Yield: About 3 cups

REFERENCES

Recent research supporting the benefits of a diet rich in fruits, vegetables, whole grains, beans, nuts and other seeds:

~ R Ahmed, I Segal, H Hassan. Fermentation of dietary starch in humans. American Journal of Gastroenterology, 2000, Volume 95, Issue 4, pp. 1017-1020.

~ DP Speechly, R Buffenstein. Appetite dysfunction in obese males: evidence for role of hyperinsulinaemia in passive overconsumption with a high fat diet. European Journal of Clinical Nutrition, 2000, Volume 54, Issue 3, pp. 225-233.

~ SJ Ley, CC Horwath, JM Stewart. Attention is needed to the high prevalence of vitamin D deficiency in our older population. New Zealand Medical Journal, 1999, Volume 112, Issue 1101, pp. 471-472.

~ S SarlioLahteenkorva, A RIssueanen, J Kaprio. A descriptive study of weight loss maintenance: 6 and 15 year follow-up of initially overweight adults. International Journal of Obesity, 2000, Volume 24, Issue 1, pp. 116-125.

~ ND Barnard, AR Scialli, P Bertron, D Hurlock, K Edmonds, L Talev. Effectiveness of a low-fat vegetarian diet in altering serum lipids in healthy premenopausal women. American Journal of Cardiology, 2000, Volume 85, Issue 8, pp. 969-972.

~ FB Hu, EB Rimm, MJ Stampfer, A Ascherio, D Spiegelman, WC Willett. Prospective study of major dietary patterns and risk of coronary heart disease in men. American Journal of Clinical Nutrition, 2000, Volume 72, Issue 4, pp. 912-921

~ S Liu, JE Manson, IM Lee, SR Cole, CH Hennekens, WC Willett, JE
Buring. Fruit and vegetable intake and risk of cardiovascular dis-
ease: the Women's Health Study. American Journal of Clinical
Nutrition, 2000, Volume 72, Issue 4, pp. 922-928.

~ LE Spieth, JD Harnish, CM Lenders, LB Raezer, MA Pereira, SJ
Hangen, DS Ludwig. A low-glycemic index diet in the treatment
of pediatric obesity. Archives of Pediatrics & Adolescent Medicine,
2000, Volume 154, Issue 9, pp. 947-951

~ SM Liu, JE Manson, MJ Stampfer, FB Hu, E Giovannucci, GA
Colditz, CH Hennekens, WC Willett. A prospective study of
whole-grain intake and risk of type 2 diabetes mellitus in US
women. American Journal of Public Health, 2000, Volume 90, Issue
9, pp. 1409-1415.

~ PR Conlin, D Chow, ER Miller, LP Svetkey, PH Lin, DW Harsha, TJ
Moore, FM Sacks, LJ Appel. The effect of dietary patterns on
blood pressure control in hypertensive patients: Results from the
Dietary Approaches to Stop Hypertension (DASH) trial.
American Journal of Hypertension, 2000, Volume 13, Issue 9, pp.
949-955.

~ LM Resnick, S Oparil, A Chait, RB Haynes, P KrisEtherton, JS Stern,
S Clark, S Holcomb, DC Hatton, JA Metz, M McMahon, FX
PiSunyer, DA McCarron. Factors affecting blood pressure respons-
es to diet: The vanguard study. American Journal of Hypertension,
2000, Volume 13, Issue 9, pp. 956-965

~ WE Connor. Importance of n-3 fatty acids in health and disease.
American Journal of Clinical Nutrition, 2000, Volume 71, Issue 1,
Suppl. S, pp. 171S-175S.

~ TAB Sanders. Polyunsaturated fatty acids in the food chain in Europe. American Journal of Clinical Nutrition, 2000, Volume 71, Issue 1, Suppl. S, pp. 176S-178S.

~ PM KrisEtherton, DS Taylor, S YuPoth, P Huth, K Moriarty, V Fishell, RL Hargrove, GX Zhao, TD Etherton. Polyunsaturated fatty acids in the food chain in the United States. American Journal of Clinical Nutrition, 2000, Volume 71, Issue 1, Suppl. S, pp. 179S-188S.

~ M Sugano, F Hirahara. Polyunsaturated fatty acids in the food chain in Japan. American Journal of Clinical Nutrition, 2000, Volume 71, Issue 1, Suppl. S, pp. 189S-196S

~ MT McGuire, RR Wing, JO Hill. The prevalence of weight loss maintenance among American adults. International Journal of Obesity, 1999, Volume 23, Issue 12, pp. 1314-1319.

~ AP Simopoulos. Essential fatty acids in health and chronic disease. American Journal of Clinical Nutrition, 1999, Volume 70, Issueue 3, Suppl. S, pp. 560S-569S.

~ SM Liu, WC Willett, MJ Stampfer, FB Hu, M Franz, L Sampson, CH Hennekens, JE Manson. A prospective study of dietary glycemic load, carbohydrate intake, and risk of coronary heart disease in US women. American Journal of Clinical Nutrition, 2000, Volume 71, Issue 6, pp. 1455-1461

~ M Noakes, PM Clifton. Changes in plasma lipids and other cardio-vascular risk factors during 3 energy-restricted diets differing in total fat and fatty acid composition. American Journal of Clinical Nutrition, 2000, Volume 71, Issue 3, pp. 706-712

~ D Li, A Sinclair, A Wilson, S Nakkote, F Kelly, L Abedin, N Mann, A Turner. Effect of dietary alpha-linolenic acid on thrombotic risk factors in vegetarian men. American Journal of Clinical Nutrition, 1999, Volume 69, Issue 5, pp. 872-882.

~ FB Hu, MJ Stampfer, JAE Manson, EB Rimm, A Wolk, GA Colditz, CH Hennekens, WC Willett. Dietary intake of alpha-linolenic acid and risk of fatal ischemic heart disease among women. American Journal of Clinical Nutrition, 1999, Volume 69, Issue 5, pp. 890-897.

RECOMMENDED BOOKS

~ Mirkin, Gabe, M.D., **Fat Free, Flavor Full**, with Diana Rich Mirkin, Little, Brown and Company, February, 1995

~ Mirkin, Gabe, M.D., **The 20/30 Fat and Fiber Diet Plan**, with Barry Fox and Diana Rich Mirkin, Harper Resource, 1998

~ Anderson, Jean and Barbara Deskins, **The Nutrition Bible**, William Morrow, 1997

~ Erasmus, Udo, **Fats that Heal, Fats that Kill**, Alive Books, 1999

~ Sizer, Frances and Eleanor Whitney, **Nutrition Concepts and Controversies**, West Wadsworth, 1997.

USEFUL WEB SITES

~ Dr. Gabe Mirkin on Health, Fitness and Nutrition
http://www.drmirkin.com
Supporting materials for the Good Food Book plus hundreds of reports to help you maintain a healthy lifestyle and understand medical breakthroughs.

~ American Institute for Cancer Research
http://www.aicr.org
Research updates and useful free publications.

~ Nutrition News Focus
http://www.nutritionnewsfocus.com
A free e-mail newsletter to help you interpret news stories on nutrition, from Wayne State University.

~ USDA Food Composition Data
http://www.nal.usda.gov/fnic/foodcomp/Data/index.html
Searchable data on 82 nutrients in more than 6,200 foods.

~ Center for Science in the Public Interest
http://www.cspinet.org
Publishers of Nutrition Action Newsletter; the web site has many articles online.

~ The Merck Manual
http://www.merck.com/pubs/mmanual_home/
Searchable text of the home version of this basic health reference.

~ Get Healthy Shop
http://www.gethealthyshop.com
Source for the whole grains cooker mentioned on page 98.

~ American Heart Association
http://www.americanheart.org
Education and information on fighting heart disease and stroke.

~ American Diabetes Association
http://www.diabetes.org
Comprehensive diabeties information, prevention and treatment.

RECIPE INDEX

ABOUT THE AUTHORS

Gabe Mirkin, M.D., hosts a daily call-in health talk show which has been on the air for more than 20 years. He is a practicing physician, board-certified in four specialties; and trained at Harvard, Baylor, Massachusetts General and Johns Hopkins Hospital. Dr. Mirkin has written eight books, 16 scientific textbook chapters, and chapters for both the physicians' and home editions of The Merck Manual. He has served as daily fitness commentator for CBS radio since 1978.

Diana Rich Mirkin, Director of Dr. Gabe Mirkin's Fat Free Clinic in Kensington, Maryland, has taught thousands of people how to make fruits, vegetables, whole grains and beans taste delicious. She is co-author with her husband of *The 20/30 Fat and Fiber Diet Plan*, *Fat Free, Flavor Full*, and *The Whole Grains Cookbook*. She appears on **The Dr. Gabe Mirkin Show** each Friday to answer questions about food and nutrition.

The Dr. Gabe Mirkin Show is syndicated in the United States and Canada. For a list of radio stations, visit www.drmirkin.com or send a self-addressed, stamped envelope to Box 10, Kensington, Maryland 20895.

TABLE OF CONTENTS